AGE-DEFYING, SOUL INSPIRED, PLANT-BASED COOKING

Gwendolyn Flynn

To your health!
Sally & Doug
Enjoy the read

Printed in the United States of America
First Printing, 2016
ISBN 978-152-034-8605

Cover Design by Jaclyn Hsiung
Book Design by Jaclyn Hsiung and Megan McCullough
Author photography: Habib KJ West

Gwendolyn J Flynn, Publisher
17522 Sherman Way
Van Nuys, CA 91406

gwenflynn@att.net

* * *

This book is lovingly dedicated to my grandchildren Malik and Jaliyah. Always trust your instincts. May you be forever curious, hungering only for knowledge. Be fearless in questioning what is, and fearless in seeking what's possible.

* * *

Table of Contents

Prologue

I might be considered a "foodie," although not hardcore. My love of food is clear. I love to eat it and love to cook it. I have strong opinions of the foods I like and don't like. I wouldn't say that I am snobbish about food. However, my tolerance of ill-prepared, unwholesome, sloppily-served food is extremely low. When my interest in cooking began, I can't say for sure. My mother was an okay cook, but I liked my aunt's cooking better, probably because of its novelty in the beginning. Only occasionally did I get to experience my aunt's cooking. My mother's cooking was what I was exposed to every day—until she died a few months after my eighth birthday. She was 41. My whole world changed.

There was no more doting, loving, nurturing mother. Because father wasn't in the picture, my two younger sisters and I were reared by my aunt and uncle. Aunt Ida was our aunt by marriage—married to my mother's brother Joe. Uncle cooked too. They were the ones who helped shape my interest in food and, by example, taught me how to cook.

This book is a product of my desperation. My body, at age 60, started to turn against me. I developed food allergies—peanuts, certain shellfish, even wheat. I began to experience high blood pressure, high cholesterol and overweight health conditions. As we've all heard, aging isn't for wimps. I developed a fibroid-like tumor near my kidney that is usually found only in the uterus of child-bearing age women. I am post-menopausal, well past having babies. And I no longer have a uterus—I had a partial hysterectomy years ago to remove a group of grapefruit-sized fibroid tumors. Yet a fibroid-like tumor grew. I learned that such tumors were fed by blood and hormones. While I still produce hormones, I no longer produce high levels of hormones, and since there was no evidence of the tumor connected to blood vessels and capillaries, it must be fed by other hormones I reasoned. Could these hormones come from the growth-hormones injected into the animals I eat? With the history of heart disease in my family, I gave up pork long ago and then removed red meat from my diet. By this time I ate mainly poultry and poultry products like turkey bacon, turkey sausage, ground turkey, and chicken. Not trusting labels, I decided to stop eating poultry as well—whether grass-fed, growth hormone free or not. No meat, period. I didn't just stop there. I decided to not eat any animal products including dairy—cheese, milk and eggs with the exception of egg whites. I stay away from starchy carbohydrates like bread, potatoes, rice and pasta except when I need to exert large amounts of energy for exercise or strenuous work. In those instances, I eat carbohydrates to sustain these activities. I felt moved to not just adopt this new diet but to learn more about it. I resumed research begun long ago.

Early in life I came to mistrust the medical community, particularly doctors trained in Western medicine. The early death of my mother contributed to the mistrust. I only remember her going to the hospital in the middle of one night and never coming back. As you can imagine, that experience left an indelible impression. Eventually my strong distrust of doctors moderated. I began reading books by doctors Andrew Weil, whom I consider to be the modern day father of the "food as medicine" approach and Joel Fuhrman, a medical doctor and author. Both are Western-trained physicians who have adopted an Eastern healing philosophy. The Eastern approach to medicine embraces practices that largely focus on illness prevention, and considering holistic approaches to healing rather than treatment and management of disease conditions. What one eats plays a significant role in that equation. This treatment of the whole person—body, mind, spirit/soul made perfect sense to me.

In my twenties and thirties I tried vegetarianism as a way to address what I thought were food allergies. I knew instinctively that eating more fruits and vegetables was healthier for me. My research continued. I have a library full of vegetarian cookbooks acquired in the 1970s and '80s. I combined research with vegetarian practice. However, practicing vegetarianism didn't last. It was short-lived because the recipes were tasteless and used ingredients unfamiliar or unavailable to me. The ingredients I use in this book are for the most part common, readily available, relatively inexpensive, and flavorful. I abandoned research for a time and relied on intuition.

Following my instincts about my personal health and healing isn't unusual or new. There was a time in this country when people of color, like me, had to rely on intuition and knowledge passed down through generations when it came to healing. We were prohibited and excluded from hospital treatment—specifically those of us who lived in the southern United States. Out of necessity, we developed our own potions, salves, and elixirs from natural, plant-based products like aloe, mustard seed, herbs and spices that we grew. Our ancestors knew what foods to eat or apply to cure ailments. I called on these close-to-the-land sensibilities of those who came before me and my own intuition to create the recipes in this book.

I agonized over the book title. I didn't want to use the term "vegetarian," which has different meanings for different individuals, and doesn't accurately reflect my dietary choices. While I eat plant-based food, I also still eat seafood other than shellfish, and egg whites. I've learned that this select diet is called pescatarianism. A pescatarian is defined as *one whose diet includes fish but no other meat*. But I thought this little known term might be a bit intimidating as part of a book title and I didn't want to scare off the curious reader.

Because this book is more than a cookbook, I wanted a title that reflected that aspect. The book contains pieces of my life that give insight into my connection to food and how I came to this plant-based diet. It also contains information about the effects of food on the human body and other relevant factual information. What emerged is the current title, **Age-Defying, Soul Inspired, Plant-Based Cooking**. Age-defying because I'm told I don't look my age. While much of that is genetics, I attribute a good portion of youth-retention to what I put into and how I treat my body. Soul inspired because for me, cooking comes from the heart and your senses, not from the head necessarily. When I'm cooking, I rely on what moves me, what has influenced me over time. It is an intangible emotional feeling I get when I cook that strives towards fulfillment and taste richness in my recipes for the diner's total meal enjoyment. The food must taste, smell, and look good in addition to making you feel good eating it and thereafter. I don't allow myself to be restricted by convention when it comes to food texture and flavor combinations. While the recipes have measurements for the ingredients, I don't hold strictly to those measurements. You shouldn't either. The amount of seasoning and ingredients are approximations according to taste. For me cooking is not a rigid, limiting science. It is another expression of one's taste preferences, experiences, background, personality, and love. Anyone with a soul can become a good cook. I'm sure all cooks can relate to that definition of soul inspired cooking.

What I share here is food-related information learned over time that has worked for me. If it works for me, there may be something in it that works for you too. The book combines innate, anecdotal knowledge, and some wisdom with facts and practice-based evidence. I invite you to try it with the precaution that you first consult with your healthcare provider before adopting any significant change that affects your health.

Brief Family Health History & Food

I am an African-American woman who was born and grew up in Rochester, New York. Rochester sits on Lake Ontario between Buffalo on the west and Syracuse on the east in upstate New York. The city was best known as headquarters to Eastman Kodak Company, the former leader in camera and film production.

Longevity isn't a family trait. I mentioned the early death of my mother from a kidney ailment; however, my maternal family has a history of heart disease and cancer. My mother was the eldest of three and the only girl. Her middle brother had his first heart attack while in his 30s. His eldest daughter, my first cousin, died of a massive heart attack at age 41. My mother's youngest brother, a heavy smoker, died of lung cancer in his 40s. My maternal grandmother died in her mid-50s. The cause of her death is unknown to me. Suffice it to say, I've witnessed the early demise of enough blood relatives from preventable, often diet-related disease and lifestyle conditions to conclude a healthy diet and lifestyle are necessary for me if I hope for a long life.

I was the odd one in my family. They all looked at me as being a bit strange. When I lived on my own in the early 1970s, I bought food from the food coop. In those days it was in the part of Rochester where all the artsy, bohemian types lived. I wasn't necessarily artsy, but I somehow identified with them and lived in that community for a time. I ate unusual, strange-looking things like bean sprouts, and tofu, rarely part of African American cuisine at the time. My family viewed those new food items they heard me talk about with raised eyebrows. *"What is she into now?"* some would whisper behind my back; others would question me to my face. They didn't know how to take me. I didn't quite fit any mold or label—not a hippy or strongly committed Black National. Although I leaned towards Black Nationalism—attracted to its political ideology of self-determination that included the politics of food—I pretty much marched to my own drum. My family and friends would humor me by listening to me talk about the connection between food and health, but wouldn't go as far as trying it. They would say *this is rabbit food and I'm not a rabbit. You can't expect me to eat that.* With this book, I'm hoping those who can identify with my story will return to the close-to-the-land orientation of our forefathers and mothers and give eating food predominately "picked, rather than slaughtered" a try for improved health and a better quality of life. I found a way to improve the flavor and texture of plant-based meals swapping out animal products. These recipes have brought me back to good health— my weight is reduced, my blood pressure has decreased to where my doctor has lowered my medication. My goal is to be completely free of medication. My cholesterol is down. As of this writing, the fibroids have not returned. A CT Scan one year after my surgery shows "no recurrence of a mass," according to my doctor. I hope to introduce you to new ingredients, inspire you to try new cooking methods. I will have accomplished my intent if you are exposed to different ingredient combinations or flavors that encourage you to experiment and trust your instincts.

Introduction

Food: The Nexus of Social Interaction

Because food is necessary to function and we humans tend to be social, food has always been the key element around which our interactions revolve. When was the last time you attended an event or an informal gathering and no food was present? We invite friends and co-workers for a meal, whether it's breakfast, lunch or dinner. Sporting events always involve food—from the non-professional end-of-season banquets for volunteer youth sports to the National Football League Super Bowl parties. Social events from the time even before we're born—baby showers, to the time we die—funeral re-passé and every event in between, include food. Those of us involved in community organizing know to promote free food on material publicizing the event to guarantee good attendance if not a packed house.

On some level of our collective consciousness, we know that food is necessary for our survival, but we never think about how it contributes to the operation of our bodies and mind. Instead we concentrate on how it looks, tastes and the ease to obtain it. This has led to the popularity of highly processed convenience foods to the detriment of our health.

It is also interesting to note the changing trends in the types of food we have eaten over the years as a piece of the American culture. In the 1950s and '60s we were eating lots of food heavily-laden with mayonnaise—potato, macaroni, and tuna salads for example. They were and still are a main-stay at picnics and parties. In the 1970s cheese ruled—cheese fondue, cheese logs, port wine cheese could be found at parties if not one or the other, in combination. In the 1980s and '90s our food started to lighten up. We used oil and vinegar on our salads, and wraps emerged as an alternative to sandwiches.

These food trends have brought about changes in food preparation—particularly for some racial and ethnic family traditions and customs. I grew up in an African American household. Although born and raised in the northeast, most of the food in my household was prepared using southern, specifically southeast recipes and cooking methods of my mother who was born in South Carolina and later my aunt. With the evolution of food trends, we changed from using lard/shortening for frying to using vegetable oil instead. We hadn't yet moved from frying to baking, but that would come.

Not only are the times we live in trending towards lighter fare, but growing research supports increasing fresh, wholesome plant-based foods in our diets to achieve optimum health and better quality of life as we age. Let's face it, we're all aging. Baby-boomers, a demographic I'm a part of, are reaching senior citizen age. We number just under 77 million in the United States.[1] We can no longer effectively process the foods we ate in our youth as part of our American culture or family tradition. Because we are living longer than the generation before us, we need to eat nutritiously to guard against compromising our health and lifestyle as we grow older. There's growing research on the population that follows us, which indicates they will be the first generation to have a shorter lifespan than their parents due to obesity and other food-related chronic diseases. If you fall into Generation X aka Gen X demographic, you will need to pay attention to the health forecasting and consider the ideas outlined in this book. Even though you may feel invincible, what you do in your life now impacts your future.

These ideas led me to write this book and spark a dialogue on another approach to food that nourishes, satisfies, and contributes to a healthier life.

Now that you have the context and background for how the idea for this publication came to be, here's what you can expect of the content.

---

1   K. Pollard, et. Al - Population Reference Bureau. Just How Many Baby
     Boomers Are There? Updated April, 2014.
     www.prb.org/Publications/Articles/2002...: Retrieved 5/3/2015.

What's Between The Covers

This book will speak to the home cook, but it is not your ordinary cookbook. Along with flavorful plant-based recipes accompanied by vivid photos of mouth-watering dishes, you will find documented information or information on the food/health connection that has been successfully applied. I refer to this information as fact/practice-based and it serves as a reminder of how food benefits us beyond satiating hunger and satisfying taste.

There are practical reasons for eating, not the least of which is to provide fuel for our bodies. Some foods, have medicinal benefits that are better than synthetic drugs—better because there are no side effects. I am not a physician and offer no medical advice. For that you should consult your medical practitioner. I hope the facts presented are enough to whet your appetite for further study. I provide endnotes of citations, references, and resources.

I don't delve too deeply into the ethical aspects of plant-based foods. That is a subject for another book.

I am not a chef. It is fair to describe me as a home cook with more than 50 years of experience in family food preparation. This book is written from that perspective. Along with the recipes and fact/practice-based health information, there's guidance on what supplies and tools I find useful to perform best in the kitchen. Although written with the home cook in mind, there is information that benefits the seasoned cook new to the plant-based orientation. There's information about the use of food processors versus manual chopping, mincing, and grinding. For some of us it doesn't feel like cooking if we aren't using a knife on something. But the kitchen of today eliminates the time it takes for manual labor with relatively inexpensive small appliances and gadgets.

I also offer cooking tips on various subjects. Tips range from spices that aid in relieving inflammation to the most efficient way to cook using beans. There is information on the use of sodium and foods that naturally contain it. Many of the ingredients for the recipes are natural and homemade. However, a few recipes include the use of bottled, processed products for the sake of convenience.

Sprinkled in the mix of information and recipes are stories about me, my family and experiences that contributed to my food-related opinions and practices. A television cooking personality recently stated that TV chef/cooks are all storytellers. I will broaden that idea and state that storytelling through food is true for those of us who don't cook before cameras as well. We all have food-related stories we can tell. It is that notion that became the impetus for this book and the recipes presented.

I begin with fact/practice-based health and nutrition information to provide background on the food/health connection.

Part 1

Food as Medicine

Let food be thy medicine and medicine be thy food.
~ Hippocrates

In my research, I discovered a school of thought promoted throughout history that experienced a resurgence in the 1980s. Dr. Andrew Weill and others espoused that the nutrients in food can support our health and well-being. The University of Minnesota's Center for Spirituality & Healing and The Center for Mind-Body Medicine (CMBM) both advance this idea. The University of Minnesota's Center for Spirituality & Healing was founded in 1995. Its mission is to enrich health and well being by providing exemplary inter-professional education, conducting rigorous research, delivering innovative engagement programs and advancing integrative models of care.[2] The Center for Mind-Body Medicine (CMBM), founded in 1991, combines evidence-based modern science, wise tradition, and human connection to create a powerful new medicine centered on self-care.[3]

The food as medicine philosophy and approach have been part of the alternative medicine movement from the beginning. While controversial in some circles, continuing discourse, growing evidence and independent study of the subject is moving the approach from the realm of alternative to mainstream. It is offered here with the

2   www.csh.umn.edu Retrieved 5/10/2015.
3   www.cmbm.org Retrieved 5/10/2015.

suggestion to the reader to conduct further study to judge for yourself the validity of the philosophy and practices.

Healing Properties of the Human Body

Dr. Weill writes in his book, *8 Weeks to Optimum Health*, "the healing system is a functional system of the body not a structural component like the nervous system or musculoskeletal system. Western medicine focuses mainly on structure." The immune system is a component of the healing system. Dr. Weill asserts that treatment can activate healing and remove obstacles to healing but the cause of all cures is the healing system (pages 17, 18).

In his forward to Dr. Fuhrman's book, Eat to Live, Dr. Mehmet Oz, a cardiovascular surgeon, references the body's healing ability as he writes in part, "I have become convinced that the most overlooked tool in our medical arsenal is harnessing the body's own ability to heal through nutritional excellence."

Given these assertions, the inference is with proper nutrients our bodies are capable of healing themselves from attacks and invasion. Cell regeneration repairs damaged cells and tissue, and generally protects the body from harmful organisms.

It is widely believed, but elevated principally in the world of alternative medicines, that the human body supported by proper nutrition has a natural ability to heal itself. For example, when you cut your finger you don't have to do anything but keep the wound clean, provided there are no other illnesses, for the cut to heal. After conducting a search for scientific evidence to support this belief, nothing conclusive was found. Unfortunately alternative medicine is, as the term indicates, just that and not recognized by the mainstream medical profession. Other than offering up examples of wounds that heal from minor cuts and scrapes, there's nothing in the literature to demonstrate concretely that when the body is significantly damaged as in a car wreck with bone and tissue damage as well as blood loss, it will automatically activate regenerative mode like super-heroes in the movies and regrow limbs. However, there is expanding information on the connection between healing from preventable diet-related disease and proper nutrition.

Eastern Medicine and Healing

When diet is wrong, medicine is of no use.
When diet is correct, medicine is of no need.
~ Ayurvedic Proverb

Ayurveda is a Sanskrit word meaning the science of life. It is interpreted by certain cultures as harmony between body, mind and spirit—holistic.[4] When that harmony is disrupted, illness and disease sets in. The world cultures that embrace this concept are East Indian, Asian, Chinese, and Japanese. Countries along the Mediterranean identify this idea with a certain "diet."[5] It is not a specific diet but collection of eating habits traditionally followed by people of Greece, Crete, Southern France and parts of Italy. In India, Ayurveda has evolved into a healthcare system.[6]

A National Institutes of Health-AARP study published in the 2007 Archives of Internal Medicine provides strong evidence of the health benefits of practicing Ayurveda lifestyle including diet. Patterns of reduced risk of death due to cardiovascular disease and cancer were found.

Another study, Lyon Diet/Heart Study of 1988 found that with adoption of a Mediterranean diet there was reduced incidence of a second heart attack or heart related deaths among 605 men and women who survived a first heart attack. Two and a half years later the study was discontinued due to compelling evidence of the health benefits.[7]

The collection of eating habits known as a Mediterranean Diet includes:

- Abundance of natural, whole, fresh plant foods
- Whole grain, high-fiber breads, cereal and rice
- Fatty fish
- Dairy products (limited)
- Olive oil

---

4   University of Minnesota, Center for Spirituality and Healing.
5   www.webmd.com › ... › Health & Balance Guide
6   University of Minnesota, Center for Spirituality and Healing.
7   www.takingcharge.csh.umn.edu. Retrieved 11/29/2014.

- High quality vinegars
- Legumes
- Herbs – fresh and dried.[8]

It's common knowledge that consuming chicken soup will help the body heal if not guard against cold and flu-like symptoms. Before I became a pescatarian, whenever I felt a cold coming on—the usual fatigue, sometimes light-headedness, slight fever symptoms, I would make a pot of broth-based soup with fresh ingredients. It was the warmth of the soup broth in combination with protein (beans or nuts—chicken isn't necessary) and vegetables—celery, onion, and carrots—mirepoix that helped flush the cold bug from my body and support the blood cells that combat foreign intruders. Within a day or so, the cold symptoms would disappear. Hot broth-based soups are the classic examples of food as medicine which most everyone can embrace. If you can accept that this works, it isn't too much of a stretch to believe that other foods have a similar healing capability.

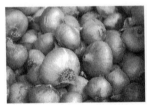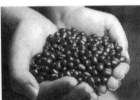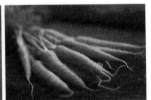

Your Body is a Temple

Most religions teach the concept that your body is a temple to hold sacred. For me that means we are not to put anything into our body or knowingly expose it to what will do it harm. When we do so unknowingly, the body will automatically defend itself against the invader. Our bodies do this without regard to moral, ethical judgment, or societal norms. Our physical bodies have no conscience. I remember when I was trying to smoke cigarettes in my late teens to early twenties to fit in with everyone around me at the time, my first inhaled puff, was immediately coughed out; rejected by my body chemistry. It

---

8   The University of Minnesota, Center for Spiritual Healing: Taking Charge of Your Health & Well-Being, The Mediterranean Diet, www.takingcharge.csh.umn.edu/mediterranean-diet. Retrieved January 2015

signaled that smoking wasn't good for me. I never became a smoker. In a similar way food not good for us can cause a reaction. It may not be as immediate as smoking was for me, but a reaction nonetheless. For example, too much sugar can cause skin blemishes, no matter what your age. Conversely, food that is good for you can cause positive reactions. Notice how you feel after eating. You may have more energy, and can think clearly. Or, depending on the amount you eat and what it was, you may feel sluggish, sleepy and unfocused. Pay attention to what your body tells you. After my surgery, I added to my prayer before eating *"...and heal my body."* Adding this to my prayer giving thanks for my food has become the following: *thank you for the food I'm receiving to nourish and heal my body and feed my mind.* This addition has made me more thoughtful about what I put in my body. It is a subtle reminder to treat my body like the temple it is.

Although there are references to food and spiritual connection as part of the holistic approach to health, you don't have to subscribe to any religion to adopt plant-based cooking. It is reasonable to expect this book to provide fact/practice-based information as necessary to spark discussion and your own curiosity.

I was born with a heart murmur, which means that along with my heartbeat, an unusual sound can be heard. You couldn't hear it with the naked ear, only with a stethoscope. Doctors predicted, I would grow out of it. As a preschooler, I had respiratory problems. Because of these conditions, my mother became very concerned when I caught a cold. It would usually settle in my lungs. As much as she was concerned, she didn't take me to the doctor, probably because of the expense. Instead, she drew from old home remedies and gave me honey and lemon to swallow for my sore throat then made a "mustard plaster" to lay on my chest. Mustard plaster demonstrates that food doesn't have to be ingested to benefit the body temple.

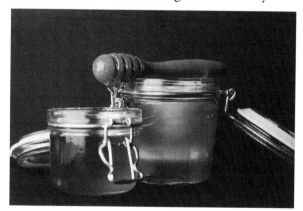

The mustard plaster consisted of a plain cotton cloth, slathered with mustard seed and flour mixed in water to form a paste. She would lay the mustard plaster on my chest. I remember feeling a sting from it. She comforted me by saying it would draw out the phlegm from my chest to help improve my breathing. I had to lie still on my back until I went to sleep. In the meantime, my mother placed a steaming pot of hot water near my bed which acted as a vaporizer. Within a day or so, my throat was no longer sore, my chest cleared, and I was breathing better.

These are my early examples of the use of food to aid the healing process. Bet if you examined your family history, you will find some home remedies of your own involving food.

It would help to be reminded how food is used by our bodies.

How The Body Processes or Metabolizes Food

In the introduction to the self-help guide Prescription for Nutritional Healing by James Balch, MD, and Phyllis Balch, CNC, they write, "think of the body as being composed of millions of tiny little engines. Some of these engines work in union, some work independently; they all are on call twenty-four hours a day. In order for the engines to work right, they require specific fuels. When the type of fuel given is the wrong blend, the engine will not perform to its maximum capacity. When the fuel is of a poor grade, the engine may sputter and hesitate, creating a loss of power. When the engine is given no fuel, it will stop. For us, much of the fuel we give our engines comes directly from the things we eat." Our bodies are the engines, food is our fuel. Food fuels our bodies and mind in the same way gasoline fuels our cars. A physician who specializes in care of diabetic patients used to say we put high octane, or the best gas in our expensive luxury cars, but when it comes to ourselves, we put cheap, or poor grade, low-nutrient food into our bodies and expect it to operate at its optimum. Something is wrong with those priorities.

According to WebMD and in its simplest description, our digestive system is designed to turn food into the energy our body needs to function and survive. Our digestive system is composed of about nine different parts. Beginning with the **mouth**, digestion starts when food enters it. Chewing mixes food with saliva that breaks the food into easily digested pieces. This starts the process of breaking down food into a form our body can absorb. The pieces then enter the **throat** and onto the **esophagus** for swallowing. The esophagus delivers the food to the stomach. The **stomach** acts like a mixer and grinder. It secretes acid and enzymes that continues the food breakdown process.

When it leaves the stomach, food has the consistency of a liquid or paste as it moves into the **small intestine**. The small intestine has three segments. It uses enzymes released by the **pancreas** and bile from the **liver** that continues the breakdown process. Bile aids in the digestion of fat and eliminates waste products from the blood. Other parts of the small intestine are responsible for the absorption of nutrients into the bloodstream. The **gallbladder** also plays a role in the secretion of bile. Once the nutrients have been absorbed, and the leftover liquid has passed through the small intestine, what remains of the food is moved into the **colon**.[9] At this point, it is ready for elimination from the body. The time it takes for this process or transit time varies and is determined by several factors, including the type and amount of food, age, gender and ethnicity.[10]

At a yoga retreat, while directing us to move our torso to help digestion and the movement of food through our bodies, the instructor stated that **trouble starts when food stays in our bodies too long.** Over the years I have heard that stated in different ways from different sources. Drs. Andrew Weill, Joel Fuhrman, and Memet Oz are all proponents of eating plenty of fiber. Fiber helps move food efficiently through our system. I've also heard that we adults should eliminate or move our bowels almost as often as babies. It wasn't until the yoga instructor made that statement that the puzzle pieces all came together for me. I share this with you now for you to examine for yourself. The recipes in this book all include plant-based fibrous ingredients. The recipes should facilitate food transit time and contribute to frequent waste elimination. Don't be afraid of gas and to eliminate or have a good poop several times a day. It's good for you.

We must change our perception and our relationship with food. We only think of food to satisfy our hunger. To do that it must be

9   www.webmd.com/heartburn-gerd/your-digestive-system. Retrieved 9/1/2014.
10   www.webmd.com/answers/5002406/how-long-does-it-take-for-food-to-pass-through-the-stomach-andsmall-intestine-to-the-large-intestine. Retrieved 9/1/2014.

pleasing to taste and to the eye. We never think about nutritional value. However, just like any piece of machinery, when you put junk in, junk comes out or even worse it doesn't come out. Instead it festers inside until it turns into something harmful.

Each time I see a laxative commercial on television, I shout at the screen, *EAT SOME FRUIT AND YOU WON'T NEED A LAXATIVE!* That is, of course, if you don't have a medical intestinal condition.

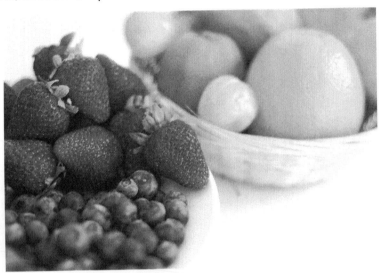

When I worked for an entertainment conglomerate in the late 1980s, there was a temporary worker or temp as we called them at the time who was transitioning from one profession to another and so was older than most temps. He was probably in his early 40s, married with two teenaged children, one headed to college. He and his family relocated to Los Angeles from the mid-West to pursue his new career. All of us in the department who knew his story thought him brave to risk changing careers at his age with the responsibilities he had. One day, he joined a group of us for lunch at a restaurant specializing in Mediterranean cuisine. It was his first experience with Mediterranean food and he asked us about our choices and what on the menu we considered good. After hearing our responses, he ordered a meal consisting mainly of greens.

Later that afternoon, he complained of having intestinal discomfort. The next day he reported having spent a good deal of the previous evening in his bathroom. The greens apparently moved his bowls more than he was used to. He was uncomfortable having so much eliminated in such a short time. I suspect he was a meat and potatoes type and didn't regularly eat enough fruits and vegetables. The lunch dominated by greens was no doubt good for him in removing waste that would have caused him problems. Had he been a regular consumer of fruits and vegetables, he wouldn't have experienced discomfort. That slight, short-term irritation is a small trade-off for clear bowels and good health.

I recently went to lunch with work colleagues. We went to a breakfast "joint" that served down home Southern-style (mostly fried) country breakfast all day. Staying true to my pescatarian practice I ordered salmon croquets, crispy brown hash potatoes, English muffins and orange juice. I was asked by the waitress if I wanted lettuce and tomato. I said yes realizing I ordered carbohydrates only since that dominated the menu. The lettuce was iceberg—composed mostly of water and little if any nutritious value. My colleagues had potatoes, eggs scrambled or over easy with grits and biscuits. Except for maybe the iceberg lettuce, there wasn't anything green or fibrous between our three plates. It all tasted very good though and the type of breakfast we were all accustomed to growing up. However, a steady diet of that, salmon croquets or not, would be hazardous to my health.

Be willing to embrace a new way of being about food. Don't hold onto types of food and ways of preparing food that no longer serve you due to cultural/family tradition or custom. A wise woman once said, "just because something is the way it is doesn't mean it always has to be that way." Lark Galloway-Gilliam, a community activist who I had the privilege of working with in transforming community systems and infrastructure to improve health, was talking about public policy. However, that adage applies to other situations too. I apply it here to personal behavior relative to food and health. In other words, don't accept a situation that exists because you think it can't be changed. Any situation can be changed. It begins with the vision that something different is possible and the willingness to make the change happen. It is my intention that the information contained here about the virtues of a plant-based diet and recipes will inspire change.

Defying Age

People have been seeking the fountain of youth forever. As we 77 million baby-boomers, age,[11] the search has never been more urgent for some of us. Scientific research on food used to slow the aging process is emerging.

Recent studies have concluded that lifestyle changes— particularly low-fat, vegetarian diets—affected telomeres that may lead to reduction in cellular aging.[12] Telomeres are small caps on the end of chromosomes that carry DNA. The Baltimore longitudinal study of aging conducted for more than fifty years concluded in 2008 that *genetics, **lifestyle** and disease processes affect the rate of aging between and within all individuals.*[13] Researchers involved with the study admitted there is still much more to learn. A small pilot study of men with prostate cancer conducted by University of California at San Francisco researchers and reported in an October 2013, *Lancet Oncology* article may be the first to show that any intervention may reduce cellular aging. Then there's the work of Dr. Roy Walford who is said to have pioneered "caloric restriction" for life extension as early as 1970s through his experiments with mice. When fed a restricted diet, the mice more than doubled their life expectancy.[14] Here again, more study is needed.

While there is no conclusive scientific evidence to support the assertion that the aging process can be delayed naturally through food, some foods have been associated with regenerative qualities for the human body. The following food groups are most often named as essential to longevity and lasting youthfulness. They are: fresh produce, beans and nuts; limited dairy; fish; and whole grains (Jaret, 2014).

---

11   U.S. Census bureau.

12   Ornish, Dean, M.D. The Lancet Oncology. Effect of comprehensive lifestyle changes on telomerase activity and telomere length in men with biopsy-proven low-risk prostate cancer; 5-year follow-up of a description pilot study; Volume 14, No. 11 p1112-1120, Oct. 2013.

13   Health and Aging; Healthy Aging: Lessons from the Baltimore Longitudinal Study of Aging. http://www.nia.nih.gov/health/publication/healthy-aging-lessons-baltimore-longitudinalstudy/ Retrieved 4.4/2014.

14   Weindruch, R., Walford, R.L, M.D. Retardation of Aging and Disease by Dietary Restriction, C.C. Thomas, Springfield, IL. 1988.

These foods in combination with adequate sleep lead one to infer that the potential is there for slowing down the aging process. In an article from the Division of Sleep Medicine at Harvard Medical School, the authors wrote under Restorative Theories, "sleep provides an opportunity for the body to repair and rejuvenate itself. In recent years, these ideas have gained support from empirical evidence collected in human and animal studies."[15]

What I Learned About Food

Food Allergies

I was one of those children in the neighborhood who always had a runny nose. I didn't know what caused it. It was considered a minor inconvenience and not significant enough to warrant a visit to the doctor. Who had money for that?! There were six of us in the household. We'd have to be bleeding profusely to see a doctor. It would be too expensive to have every ailment each of us suffered under a doctor's care. From my teens and into adulthood, I attributed my respiratory ailment to the environment, grasses, trees, etc. of my upstate New York hometown of Rochester. There the climate offers four seasons. In the spring when wildlife awakens from winter's hibernation, the air is full of pollen and other elements that wreak havoc with people like me with allergies—hated that time of year. Fall became my favorite season when the air was pollen free, plant life shedding their allergen irritating adornment, settling in for winter.

When I grew older, and moved from Rochester to the semi-arid climate of Los Angeles California, I began noticing my body reacting to other than the environment. I deduced it was the food I ate. Nose congested, sneezing, watery eyes, sometimes even aching bones were associated not with a cold, but with eating some allergy triggering food. I discovered that all the foods I loved growing up—shrimp, peanuts, and other foods caused an allergic reaction. My body would defend itself as if it were fighting off a cold or the flu. Before I pinpointed the cause, and depending on what I ingested during a week, I was always feeling like I had a cold. In that state your body automatically works to defend itself against the intruder. It is exhausting. I began to pay attention to what

15   www.healthysleep.medharvard.edu/.../benefitsofsleep/why_ do_we_sleep.
     December 18, 2007

I put in my body. I realized that food is for more than just filling your belly and pleasing to taste. Food generates energy to keep you going and reacts to your chemical make-up in a way that can benefit or harm your health. While I came to this realization about the food I eat, I was soon to discover you don't have to eat the food to have an allergic reaction.

While sitting with me in a small conference room at work, my colleagues were shelling and eating peanuts. Before long my eyes watered; soon after I became congested and began to sneeze. After a few more minutes, my throat swelled. One of my colleagues asked me if I was allergic to peanuts. I said no. Even if I were, I had not ingested any. It wasn't until I left the room to blow my nose that I got any relief. After a time away from the peanut-filled air, I could breathe again. It was then I learned I was allergic to peanuts and apparently don't have to eat them to get a reaction, but can't even be in a room with them. What a scary, revealing episode.

Because everyone's body chemistry is unique, foods respond differently to different people. The most important lesson I learned is that food shouldn't be taken for granted.

Food for the fun of it is a major food company's slogan. I believe it is also the attitude of most people. We eat some foods because they're fun to eat—popcorn, chips of all kinds, etc. We must take our food more seriously. Part of that serious attitude is to pay attention to how your body reacts to food. Be aware that some of the ailments you are experiencing might be food related. The best way to test this is through a process of elimination. Eliminate from your food intake each food product ingested one by one until you find the offending culprit.

Soy and Health

Soy is derived from soybeans also known as edamame. Soy products include soymilk, tofu, tempeh, miso, vegetarian "meat" and dairy substitutes like soy cheeses. Consuming plant food with the least amount of processing—in other words fresh, unprocessed plant food— is the ideal health supporting practice. There have been controversial and even contradictory reports on the connection between soy products and health.

Studies have shown reduced risk of fibroids, breast and colon cancer in women who consume soy due to the phytoestrogen compound in soy.[16] Phyto refers to plants.[17] The plant estrogen counters or blocks the effect of women's natural estrogen as a partial explanation.[18] A phyto-nutrient is a bioactive plant-derived compound associated with positive health effects. Soy has been shown to be effective in addressing high cholesterol, high blood pressure, prevention of heart diseases, Type 2 diabetes, asthma, and various cancers.[19]

On the other hand, soy products are high in protein. It may be prudent to avoid high concentrations of protein from any source.[20] This may increase the amount of insulin-like growth factor in the bloodstream and this compound is linked to higher cancer risk.[21]

Organic vs. Non-Organic

The eleventh edition of Merriman-Webster's Collegiate Dictionary defines "organic" as: *(1) of, relating to, or derived from living organisms; (2) of, relating to, yielding or involving food produced with the use of feed or fertilizer of plant or animal origin without employment of chemically formulated fertilizers, growth stimulants, antibiotics, or pesticides.* In other words, as relates to food, food produced using living organisms, and no chemicals. I highly recommend and endorse organically grown/produced food over non-organic. Our body chemistries are too unique and complex to guarantee there can be no effect on humans from chemically-treated food ingested over time. Although a study on the health effects of organic food published in NJAS Wageningen Journal of Life Sciences, December 2011 by M. Huber concluded "… there appeared no simple relationship between nutritional value and health effects. It is difficult therefore to draw conclusions from

16 Soy Protein Isolate and Protection Against Cancer. Thomas M. Badger, Martin J.J. Ronis, Rosalia C.M. Simmen, Frank A. Simmen, Journal of the American College of Nutrition, Vol. 24, Iss. 2, 2005.

17 Soy and Health, Physicians Committee for Responsible Medicine. www.pcrm.org/health/health-topics/soy-and-your-health. Retrieved 5.23.2015.

18 Ibid.

19 WebMD. Soy: Uses, Side Effects, Interactions and Warnings. www.wedmd.com/vitamines-supplements/ingredientmono-975-SOY.aspx? Retrieved 8.23.2015.

20 Soy and Health, Physicians Committee for Responsible Medicine. www.pcrm.org/health/health-topics/soy-and-your-health. Retrieved 5.23.2015.

21 www.nutritionfacts.org. Volume 10, September 25, 2012, Journal of Medicinal Food IGF-1 As One Stop Cancer Shops.

analytical data about the health effects of organic foods..."[22] More longitudinal research is needed.

To meet organic certification, certain standards established by the United States Department of Agriculture (USDA) for the National Organic Program must be met. For organic crops, a summary of the standards are as follows: *The USDA organic seal verifies that irradiation, sewage sludge, synthetic fertilizers, prohibited pesticides, and genetically modified organisms were not used.*[23] Organic certified agents are nationwide.

Carbohydrates or Low Carbohydrates

Carbohydrates play an essential role in the body including providing energy for working muscles, fuel for the central nervous system, enabling metabolism and preventing protein from being used as energy. It is the preferred source of energy or fuel for muscle contraction and biologic work.[24] In other words, carbohydrates are key to making the body function. If you are an athlete, carbohydrates are crucial to providing energy for optimal performance. Exertion of any kind, think exercise, also depends on energy from carbohydrates to function. Foods containing carbohydrates are grains, fruit, and milk. Vegetables have a small amount of carbohydrates.

After a carbohydrate is eaten, it is broken down into smaller units of sugar in the stomach and small intestine. These small units of sugar are absorbed in the small intestine and they enter the bloodstream where they travel to the liver. The liver converts certain sugar components into glucose. Glucose is the carbohydrate transported by the bloodstream to the various tissues and organs, including the muscles and the brain, where it will be used as energy.[25]

---

22 NJAS-Wageningen Journal of Life Sciences, Volume 58, Issues 3-4, December 2011, Page 103-109, Organic Food and Impact on Human Health: Assessing the status quo and prospects of research, M.Huber.

23 www.ams.usda.gov/AMSv1.o/NOPOgranicStandards, Retrieved 9/1/2014.

24 Carbohydrate, Role of Carbohydrate, Energy Needs, Iowa State University Extension and Outreach, Human Sciences. www.extension.iastate.edu/humanscienes/content/carbohydrate. Retrieved 1/3/2015.

25 Carbohydrate, Role of Carbohydrate, Energy Needs, Iowa State University Extension and Outreach, Human Sciences. www.extension.iastate.edu/humanscienes/content/carbohydrate. Retrieved 1/3/2015.

Most carbohydrates can be divided in two groups—simple and complex or high. An example of a simple carbohydrate is the sucrose or sugar found in candy, soda, juice, etc. Simple carbohydrates produce energy that lasts for short periods. Complex or high carbohydrates are starchy and have fiber for a larger structure and endurance. Common foods consisting of complex carbohydrates are bread, pastas and whole grains. Complex carbohydrates are most important for athletes. You hear of distance runners, college and professional football players "bulking" up on complex carbohydrates prior to an athletic event.

Low Carbohydrate Diets

A low carbohydrate diet is generally used for weight loss. Some low-carb diets may have health benefits like reducing risk factors associated with diabetes and metabolic syndrome. Metabolic syndrome is a health condition that affects one out of six people. According to the Mayo Clinic, the condition is defined as: increased blood pressure, high blood sugar level, excess waistline body fat, and abnormal cholesterol levels that occur together increasing risk of heart disease, stroke, and diabetes. The low-carb diet concept is based on the belief that decreasing carbs lowers insulin levels, which causes the body to burn stored fat for energy and ultimately leads to weight loss. Low-carb diets focus on proteins including meat, poultry, fish and eggs as well as some non-starchy vegetables.[26]

Most research on low-carb diets has lasted less than a year, so it is unclear whether there are long-term health risks associated with this type of diet.

Clearly carbohydrates are important to a healthy body. It is a matter of proportion. A low-carbohydrate diet is inconsistent with plant-based eating.

While I don't consider myself a Type A personality, I do have boundless energy. That is when I'm properly fueled with carbohydrates. When I first took on this new way of eating, I did what normally happens when we try something new, we go to extremes. For me that meant completely removing carbohydrates from my diet—no potatoes, no rice, no pasta, no bread. After a couple of days, maybe weeks, I began to feel run-down and couldn't understand why. I questioned,

---

26   Ibid.

am I working that hard? Am I not getting enough sleep? Instead of buzzing from one activity to another as normal, I had to stop and take big breaks between activities. I felt like a wet rag. Then I learned that we need carbohydrates not only for strenuous activity, but any activity. What a difference when I reintroduced potatoes, couscous and other complex carbohydrates into my meals. I felt normal again. Do not under estimate the power of carbohydrates. Trying to function without them is like being superheroes on Kryptonite.

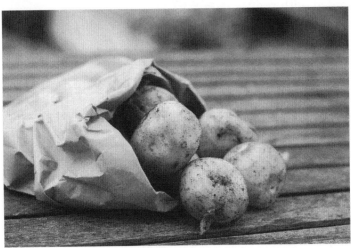

Diabetes

Diabetes is a chronic, lifelong condition that affects your body's ability to use food energy. There are three major types: Type 1, insulin dependent, was formerly called juvenile-onset diabetes because it often begins in childhood. This type of diabetes may be caused by genetic predisposition. Type 2 used to be called adult-onset diabetes. However, with the obesity epidemic, more adolescents and teenagers are developing this condition. Obesity is a risk factor for Type 2 diabetes. The third type is gestational diabetes. This condition develops in women during pregnancy. It is caused by the placenta making hormones that can lead to a build- up of blood sugar.[27] Type 2 diabetes is the most common form of diabetes, making up 95% of diabetes cases in adults. Some 26 million American adults have been diagnosed with the disease. Type 2 diabetes can be controlled with

---

27   www.wedmd.com/diabeteshealthcenter/diabetesguide. Retrieved 4/12/2015

weight management, nutrition and exercise.[28] As established above, glucose fuels cells in your body for energy. It uses the hormone insulin to take in the glucose and use it for energy. Diabetics either don't make enough insulin, or can't use the insulin they produce or a combination of both. The glucose builds up in the bloodstream. High levels of blood glucose can damage tiny blood vessels in kidneys, heart, eyes or nervous system. This damage can lead to kidney failure, heart attack, blindness and amputation of limbs. These circumstances can be prevented with proper nutrition.

Let's get ready for age-defying, soul inspired, plant-based cooking.

---

28   www.webmd.com/diabetes/type-of-diabetes-mellitus?page=1-3
      Retrieved 1/3/2015

Part 2

Prepare to Cook

What's in my Pantry

In preparation for your journey into plant-based cooking, your kitchen needs some basic food items that will enhance your eating experience. The food items I use most often are shared below. Most of you may already have them in your pantry. Some are exotic sounding spices and herbs only if you are unfamiliar with them. Don't let that stop you from trying them. You are not required to be a gourmet to enjoy them. There are other spices and herbs available, but these make frequent appearances in my dishes.

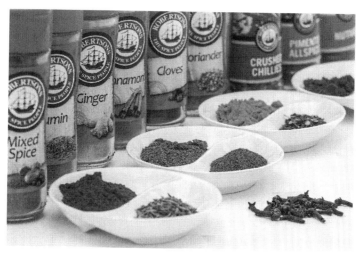

Spices

A vast array of wonderfully flavorful natural spices make plant-based dishes pop with taste. Spices are another way to reduce the need to add salt. Many of the spices listed here come fresh or dried ground. Ground is the form I use most often. None of these spices are so exotic they can't be found in any supermarket at affordable prices.

- *Turmeric* – has a peppery, slightly bitter flavor with a mild fragrance and warm color. It has the added benefit of acting as an anti-inflammatory. Inflammation contributes to bone joint problems like arthritis. Add to soups, sauces and vegetable stews like chili.

- *Nutmeg* – most cooks are familiar with this spice as an ingredient in baking. With that orientation, it will seem strange to add it to dark, leafy greens like collards. When used in this way the strong, pungent flavor of this spice reduces any bitter taste the greens might have.

- *Curry* – there are different types of curry. Some have a heat quality. I use curry powder that is mild. In addition to the indescribable unique flavor, it adds an appetite-appealing color to any dish.

- *Black pepper* – this spice is a staple in most kitchens and cuisines.

- *Dried crushed red pepper* – just the right amount gives any dish a bit of heat for added zing. I use it in Southern style greens—collards, mustard, turnips as well as cabbage, and chard.

- *Ginger* – I add this to carrots in its grated form to give the carrots a little kick. Ginger is also used to settle an upset stomach and to aid in almost any digestive circumstance.

- *Cumin* – gives pureed beans a smoky flavor. It also adds dimension to fish, dips and sauces, dressings, stews and marinades.

- *Coriander* – has a nutty, citrusy flavor with seafood, marinades and hearty dishes like stews, soups. A little goes a long way.

- *Cardamom* – has a lemony brightness yet peppery taste that works well in savory dishes and balances sweet entrees and desserts. It is related to ginger and is used as a condiment and in medicine.

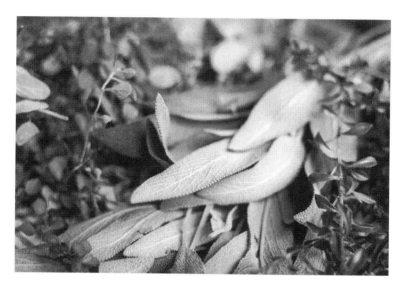

Herbs

These aromatic plants are nature's portal into flavorful dishes. All of those listed here can be home grown as potted plants or in a garden. They are all also readily available at any supermarket. They come dried, but provide the best flavor when fresh.

- *Rosemary* – Most often associated with meats, rosemary is a fine addition to any vegetable based broth, sauce, stew or soup. A little goes a long way.

- *Basil* – Enhances the flavor of tomato-based dishes like the vegetable lasagna recipe contained within.

- *Bay Leaves* – I use this with my lentil stew and chili. It has a smoky flavor. It adds richness and goes well with any soup, or stew.

- *Oregano* – Another herb that combines well with tomato-based dishes. I also like it to season fish like salmon or halibut.

- ***Mint*** – I discovered this herb adds a nice pop to salads. The herb brightens pureed beans especially garbanzo beans. It awakens the flavors of different greens.

- ***Dill*** – Most often associated with fish, dill is good in salads as well particularly in salad dressing. Add it to a lemon or oil and vinegar dressing.

- ***Chives*** – A cousin of the onion. It gives dishes a subtle onion flavor and adds a bit of color. It can be added to a variety of dishes including salads, light dressings, stews, and soups.

As I stated in the opening to this section, all of these plants can be home grown. If you have a green thumb, you may try growing your own herbs. Generally, I'm good with plants and flowers. I've had lots of success with ivies and coleus. Somehow, when it comes to edible plants like herbs, I'm a mess. For example, I tried twice unsuccessfully to grow rosemary. I've seen it growing wild in vacant lots. They appear to be a hearty herb. It has been known to take over a yard or garden because of its heartiness. How hard could it be to grow? Apparently for me, very hard. I don't strike the proper balance and have killed two rosemary plants. My lack of success doesn't mean I'm giving up. I will try again until I figure it out. If you haven't already done so, growing herbs might be your entry into home gardening. You'll have fresh picked vegetables and may save bushels of money—pun intended.

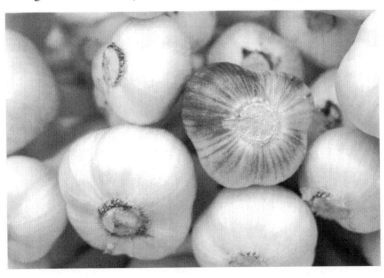

Other Pantry Must Haves

- *Garlic* – One can never have too much of this pungent root. There aren't many dishes that won't be improved with the addition of garlic. It is a known antioxidant that inhibits cancer producing free radicals. Fresh garlic is best when used no later than 7 days after purchase. It should be stored in a cool dry location. Jars of minced garlic can be refrigerated up to 14 days.

- *Scallions* – A hybrid of onion and garlic is best fresh. Store whole in a cool, dry location for up to 5 days. Cut scallions should be used no later than 3 days refrigerated in a covered container or plastic bag.

- *Onions* – Yellow, brown, red, green. Each variety has a distinct fiery flavor. Yellow onions have a sweetness when cooked. The sweetness is punctuated when caramelized. Red onions are the most potent. They have a strong aroma and are best raw. Of the onion varieties, green onions have the most subtle flavor. They store whole in a cool dry location for about 7 days. Cut, they should be refrigerated in a covered container and stored for no more than 3 days.

- *Anchovies* – These miniature fish have a concentrated fishy taste. They have a strong salty flavor. Those of us watching our sodium intake, should use them cautiously. For storage, follow the instructions on the can or jar.

- *Dried Beans* – a source of protein, and my primary protein source. Keep your favorite beans on hand. A day before I need them, I usually soak the beans for 8 hours, simmer them in vegetable broth until tender and store them in the refrigerator until I'm ready to use them. They usually keep for 3 to 5 days refrigerated. Frozen they can keep at least 14 days. There is a section on cooking with beans later in the book.

- ***Vegetable broth or stock*** – [organic, no or low sodium] I find this item incredibly invaluable to my cooking. I use the terms broth/stock interchangeably. You'll see both terms in the recipes that follow. I use the broth/stock instead of water for cooking beans, greens, quinoa, and just about everything. It gives body and a depth of flavor like nothing else.

- ***Crimini mushrooms*** – also known as baby Portobello. They have a cancer fighting property about them and have a hearty, full texture and earthy flavor. I use them liberally.

- ***Quinoa*** – a grain that can be used in place of pasta or rice. It contains loads of protein and fiber. However like rice or pasta, it is stubbornly tasteless and requires loads of added flavor.

- ***Extra Virgin Olive Oil*** – it's light, versatile for cooking and in salad dressings. It is heart friendly—in that it won't raise cholesterol. For foods that require high heat, you will need to use a different kind of oil like canola or vegetable oil. You won't find recipes like that in this book.

- ***Avocados*** – I'm lucky enough to live in the Southern California climate where avocados are plentiful. They contain good fat. Not only do I use them in salads and dips, but avocados are good for adding fat, or use as a base for soups and sauces. They have a short shelf life. If you buy them when they are solidly firm, that is no give when you press them, it may take 2-3 days to ripen at room temperature or warmer. They are ripe and ready for eating when they give when squeezed. If you don't plan to use them right away, they can be refrigerated to extend their life.

What's in my Refrigerator

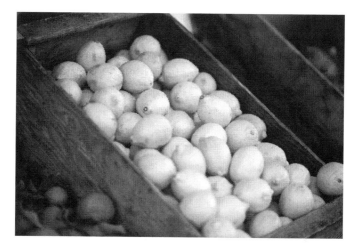

- *Non-dairy milk: almond, rice, coconut* – These non-dairy milks are among the plant-based choices available. Select the kind you like best. No need to have them all. As you can imagine, they add a creamy richness to dishes. They are fortified with calcium. There's also soy milk. However, I steer clear of soy because of warnings it may be harmful to women.

- *Lemons* – This versatile, flavor-enhancing fruit is used for fresh juice with vegetables particularly greens. The juice is also used as a base in salad dressings. Its skin can be used as a zest or peel to add brightness to a dish.

- *Egg substitute or egg whites* – I use Reddi-Egg, an egg substitute, but there are other similar products on the market. Concerned for the cholesterol contained in eggs, I opted to use egg substitutes or egg whites. Now researchers tell us that eggs aren't the culprits for cholesterol.[29] However, I continue my practice of using an egg substitute in case more research reverses that study's findings. Separating egg whites from yolks has been problematic. I don't want to waste the yolk.

---

29 http://health.gov/dietaryguidelines/2015-scientific-report,
    Released October 2015

- ***Non-dairy butter*** – I use a product called Earth Balance but there are many similar products on the market that serve as a substitute for the dairy product. They especially give sauce dishes depth. Be aware these non-dairy products do contain artificial ingredients and claim not to contain "bad" fats, but be careful of trans fats. Hydrogenated or trans fats contribute to blood cholesterol. However, I believe the potential harm from dairy products with antibiotics, growth hormones and such outweighs the concern for artificial ingredients.

The above are some of what to keep handy for meal preparation, it's certainly not everything. Because these items are for the most part fresh, and all natural, they need to be used relatively quickly, within 3 to 5 days. Except for the dried beans and spices, there isn't any need for long-term storage.

My Essential Basic Cooking Tools

In cooking these recipes, it is practical to have the tools you need and will use to perform the cooking. You can get as fancy and elaborate as you desire. Seasoned cooks can skip this section. You, no doubt, have these and more in your kitchen. For those new to cooking, below are the basic instruments you will need for cooking the recipes in this book.

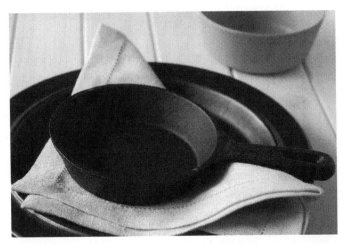

- *Pots and Pans* – 10" nonstick skillet; 1-quart, 2-quart, and 3-quart sauce pans with lids; Dutch oven—a versatile covered pan that can move from stove top to oven to table to refrigerator. Dutch ovens are generally used for dishes requiring extended cooking time. I have used a Dutch oven to cook chili, soup or to roast root vegetables. Some may find a cast iron skillet just as handy. However, I never used a cast iron skillet for any of the recipes contained in this book. A wok would be good to have for the stir-fry vegetables, but the recipes can be prepared without it.

- *Baking Dish* – A 9 X 11 shallow baking dish is invaluable to me. I use it for roasting vegetables, vegan lasagna, stuffed bell peppers and more.

- *Cooking Utensils* – To preserve your nonstick pots and pans, you can't go wrong with wooden spoons of every type—different sizes, solid, slotted, spatulas, ladles.

- *Cutlery* – For dicing, chopping, slicing for those of you who like to do it yourself, you'll need a few fundamental sharp knives. A vegetable peeler comes in handy as well.

- *Cutting Board* – Of course, you will need a cutting board on which to conduct your chopping. For sanitary reasons, I recommend easy to clean Lucite boards.

- *Food Processor(s)* – For convenience, it is nice to have a food processor available. They come in both mini and large sizes like a 9-cup capacity and are easy to use and clean.

- *Garlic crusher/mincer* – Suppose you're wondering, if I have a food processor, why would I need a garlic crush? If you buy whole garlic, there are times when you only need a small amount of garlic. These little gadgets come in handy to use efficiently.

- *Grater* – If you prefer not to use food processor, then you will need a grater. Perhaps graters of different sizes. One to grate large vegetables like cabbage for making cole slaw, and one for smaller vegetables like onion or garlic.

- ***Whisk*** – This gadget works faster than a fork in fluffing egg whites and liquids. It's handier than a mini food processor or blender for smaller quantities.

- ***Potato Masher*** – It is used for more than potatoes. It is a fairly simple way to change the texture of a food product.

When making a filling for a cabbage wrap using garbanzo beans, I pulled out my food processor for what I thought would be an easy transformation of the firm nutty bean into a roughly mashed version of itself to make a perfect filling for a cabbage leaf. It turns out, the food processor did its job too well. After just a few pulsing seconds, the beans were turned into a smooth paste. Not the texture I wanted or needed for my cabbage wrap. In my next attempt, I used a hand powered potato masher instead. I was able to reach my desired bean consistency in just a few steady, determined presses. Sometimes the new-fangled state-of-the-art gadgets take a back seat to old school know how. Now that you have your pantry and refrigerator stocked and basic cooking utensils, here are tips on cooking with beans. As a protein substitute, many of the recipes in the following pages call for beans.

Cooking with Beans

Beans are a good source of fiber and protein. Health experts believe that if you eat large amounts of fat and protein from animal sources, your risk of heart disease or certain cancers may increase.[30] Beans are a good substitute for animal protein. They add texture and flavor to any dish. I found it best to use dried beans for these recipes. While canned beans are more convenient, they contain high amounts of sodium to extend their shelf life. Most canned beans, some frozen foods and other processed food contain extra sodium. What's good for shelf life is not so good for our bodies. I recommend soaking beans in water for 5 hours or overnight. Soaking reduces cooking time, and for those of you who are worried, removes the property in beans that causes flatulence (gas). You can store soaked drained beans in an air tight container and refrigerate if you aren't using them

---

30 www.mayoclinic.org/healthy-living/weight-loss/in-depth/low-carb-diet/art-20045831?pg=1. Retrieved 1/3/2015

right away or you can cook and then store in an air tight container in the refrigerator. They will keep in the refrigerator up to 7 days. Cooking soaked beans until tender usually takes no more than 30-45 minutes depending on the bean. Cooked beans can be frozen 14 days or longer. In an on-line article entitled How Beans Help our Bones, Michael, Greger, M.D. wrote in part, "...increasing consumption of beans, legumes is universally recommended for health promotion... ." However, phytates, a naturally occurring compound found in all plant seeds like beans, grains, and nuts, is associated with mineral absorption inhibitors. To counter the inhibitors, roast, sprout or soak plant seeds to rid them of phytates and allow for mineral absorption.[31] My favorite beans are:

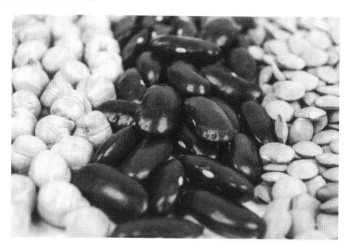

- *White Great Northern or Navy* – adds heartiness and heft to soups, and stews. The longer it's cooked, the soupier it gets. This bean is fabulous on its own too, maybe seasoned with a bit of hot sauce and cornbread on the side.

- *Garbanzo aka Chick Peas* – has a nutty texture and can be eaten alone as a snack and a protein companion in salads and of course, in main dishes or entrees.

- *Lentils* – a light bean that is good as a soup with a few added vegetables. This bean gives fullness to a dish.

---

31   www.nutritionfacts.org Retrieved 11.29.2014

- ***Red Kidney*** – a hearty bean usually used in chili and tomato-based soups and other dishes.

- ***Black*** – has a great distinctive flavor. It generally is found in Latin foods. Great in chili.

- ***Lima*** – adds body to any dish. I was first introduced to this bean as a child through succotash, a combination of lima beans and corn.

- ***Small White*** – cousin to the White Great Northern bean, it has a similar flavor. In addition to its smaller size, the other distinguishing characteristic from its cousin is it holds its shape and firm texture (unlike some of us the longer we are on earth) no matter how long it's cooked. For that reason it is the better protein choice to accompany greens or other vegetables for texture contrast. I like it as its own dish with corn bread.

- ***Black-eyed Peas*** – more of a bean than a pea. It can be used in salads and served as a side-dish. In the South eating this bean on New Year's Day is believed to bring good luck throughout the year.

Part 3

Recipes & Food-related Memories

Family Meals

It seems the best family traditions generally begin in the kitchen… is how the commercial starts to sell us on the purchase of some food product or another. It's an attention grabber because there's some truth in that statement. In most families the kitchen is the hub around which all family gatherings revolve. The kitchen is where meal preparation for all occasions takes place. It is where food customs are passed down. It is the place in many homes where families gather and food is eaten without the formality of the dining room.

It is somewhat of a novelty today, but growing up in the 60s and 70s, we ate dinner together at home in the kitchen. Unlike families today, when we ate out—usually at a fast food restaurant—it was a special occasion. There were six children. Following the death of my mother, my two sisters and I were taken in by my mother's brother and his wife. They had two children at the time with one more on the way. My aunt and uncle worked factory and post office jobs respectively. Although we didn't know it, we were probably considered the working poor with middle-class values. It was too costly to eat out regularly for a family of that size with modest income. Dinners were standardized. We could rely on a set dinner menu for each day of the week. Each selection had meat as the focal point. The pattern was as follows:

Sunday: The big meal of the week. Usually a roast of some kind of meat—beef, pork, or chicken served with potatoes and collard greens, green beans, or some other vegetable as side dishes.

Monday: Leftovers from Sunday.

Tuesday: Fried pork chops, or liver or chicken served with rice, or macaroni and cheese, cabbage, broccoli or green beans.

Wednesday: Spaghetti night. We didn't call it pasta back then. It was just spaghetti with meat sauce. The meat sauce was made with ground beef. We called it spaghetti whether it was lasagna or another form of pasta like curly-cues. It was served with a garden salad usually and at times buttered white bread. We used bread to sop up the meat sauce.

Thursday: Casserole—tuna/noodle or some other kind of tuna combination; stuffed green peppers might appear on this day.

Friday: Fish, pan fried. Although we were Presbyterian not Catholic, we always had fish on Friday. The fish of choice was porgy. It is a meaty fish regionally available in upstate New York. I could never find any when I moved west. Fish sticks would often make an appearance on Friday as a substitute for fresh fish.

Saturday: This day was reserved for more casual dinners—sloppy Joes, hot dogs and pork 'n' beans. Interestingly enough at that time, we never considered pizza a meal. It was more a snack. What a difference a couple of decades makes.

The dessert course of the meal was usually reserved for Sunday. We seldom if ever had dessert with weeknight dinner.

Learning to Cook

As a child and before this notion of food as medicine came into my awareness, I carried on family cooking traditions. There were no formal cooking lessons in our household. I learned by watching my aunt and uncle move around the kitchen preparing meals—observing pots and pans, tools, and spices used. I listened to their conversations, and tasted the results of their creations. Yes, uncle cooked too, though not often. Home Economics at school had not yet entered the picture. From the age of 11 or 12 and older, the "three big kids" (older kids age range 9-12) of six children took turns cooking meals during the week while aunt and uncle worked. There was 2 to 3 years difference in our ages with me the eldest. We each were assigned a week to cook. I remember cooking liver for one meal. To season it, we used salt and black pepper. It was floured (using a brown paper bag with flour in it), and fried in a cast iron skillet. On one particular occasion, I somehow forgot to flour the liver before placing it in the skillet with hot grease. Rookie cook's mistake.

Without the flour there was no browned coating on the cooked liver. It was just this grayish-purple hunk of meat on a plate. It didn't matter what side dishes were served with it. It was not very appealing. It is said that appearance and presentation are 90% of the dining experience. No one wanted dinner that night. It was enough to turn one off from liver, if not meat altogether.

Later on I learned that most African American kitchens, no matter where in the country we lived, stocked cans of unrefrigerated cooking grease stored not too far from the stove. It was probably a fire hazard but no one was thinking safety, only saving money. The grease was derived from shortening. Back in the day, Crisco was the shortening brand of choice used to start the cooking process in our household. Before Crisco made vegetable oil, they sold solid white shortening in tin cans. To save money, there were reused Crisco tin cans full of left-over grease—one can each for collecting grease from cooking bacon, fish, and chicken to re-use for the next fried meat. I probably used the bacon grease to fry the liver.

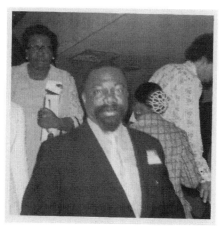

Uncle Joe and Aunt Ida, my cooking mentors, leaving Ebony Fashion Fair

Over the years, I've learned to reduce my ecological footprint by using every bit of food ingredients so that there's nothing left, which is how reusing the grease run-off may have gotten started. For economic reasons, our fore bearers had zero waste. In my plant-based cooking, I'm resurrecting that practice. For example, when I cut away the broccoli stalks from the florets, I store the stalks for use in soups or stews. The same is true for other vegetables. If I find I can't use them, I will place them in a compose bin to be used to enrich soil for growing more food. My food scraps are used in the same way.

Almighty Corn

It is one of the most versatile of vegetables and quite controversial. Without diving deeply into the many perspectives of corn including its cultural aspects, I will just discuss it as one of many common plant ingredients with health implications. As a food, corn is used to make cornmeal for cornbread and muffins and as a coating. It is an important ingredient in making the food additive, high fructose corn syrup that has become hotly debated as a contributor to obesity. High fructose corn syrup is an additive found in a substantial number of processed foods and beverages like soda, cereals, etc. Read your labels. You will be surprised to see how many food products contain corn. Know that high fructose corn syrup, while it contains "corn" in its name, is not all natural and may not be good for you.

Corn is also used in the production of ethanol discussed as a potential substitute for petroleum to fuel motored vehicles. Due to the high demand for corn, farmers and producers have found it necessary to enhance production of this commodity with genetically engineered organisms. I stay away from genetically modified organisms or GMOs as much as I can until there is conclusive evidence of no harm to human health. Where corn is concerned, I only eat what I know to be GMO free corn, if I eat it at all.

Corn is also used to make the popular breakfast cereal, cornflakes. Whether the corn used is GMO free is debatable. We ate cornflakes regularly growing up. I remember having it for breakfast on a visit to my grandmother's house in South Carolina.

BREAKFAST

To Grandmother's House We Go

We took the train from Rochester, New York to visit Grandma in Fort Mill, South Carolina. Fort Mill is a township of York County in South Carolina, but just near enough to the northern border to be considered a suburb of Charlotte, North Carolina near Rock Hill. I used to hear my mother and Uncle Joe talking about these places. The way they were discussed, I thought Fort Mill and Rock Hill were one in the same.

I must have been pre-school age, maybe 4 or just 5 years old when we traveled. I don't recall a great deal about our journey except that it was exciting to be on a train with our sandwiches and potato salad. We stopped in Washington, D.C. and visited with cousins. We replenished our travel food with fried chicken in a brown paper bag. At about 5 years old, I don't know if we brought our own food because we didn't have the money to buy it on the train or because where the trained stopped—particularly places in the South— didn't serve Negroes, as we were called at the time. The year was 1956 or so. When we arrived in Fort Mill, I'm not sure how we traveled from the train station to Grandma's house. I remember her house being in the woods. It was dark when we arrived. Walking through the dark woods was scary. The house was small, maybe three rooms. When you entered the house you were in the kitchen/living room. There was a wood-burning stove in the corner. I don't remember much color in the house. Only grays and browns. Area rugs covered the crude hardwood floor. Two bedrooms were off the kitchen/living room. What really stood out for me was learning there was no bathroom in the house. I was surprised we were in a house with no bathroom. There was a small house just behind the main house used for the toilet. An outhouse. I remember my 5 year old mind thinking how strange that was. I thought every house had a bathroom. The outhouse was smelly. I tried not to use it as much as I could during our visit.

Mother and I slept together in one of the bedrooms. The bed was cushiony, I imagined like sleeping on a cloud. The quilt warm and cozy. I must have been tired the night of our arrival. I may have quickly fallen asleep because I don't remember anything else that night. The next thing I knew it was morning. The sound of a rooster's crowing woke me up. I didn't want to get out of the warm bed. The air was crisp and stung my face. With the light of day, and standing behind the screen to the door that opened to the porch, I could see chickens roaming around the front yard. I believe there were pigs too. Grandma was in the front yard feeding the chickens some sort of corn mixture. She asked me if I wanted to feed them. I took a handful of the corn and tried to imitate her, sweeping my arm in front of me spreading the feed. I watched as the chickens gathered pecking at the feed. I remembered the **Old McDonald had a farm** song from Miss Rita's Romper Room on television and asked no one in particular, *is this a farm?* The answer was no. There was no further explanation than that. I was lucky to get an answer because at that time, children were seen but not heard.

For breakfast that morning, we had cornflakes. Cornflakes I was familiar with. Condensed milk was new to me. It was used instead of regular whole milk poured over the cereal. It was warm. The milk was too thick, too creamy, and too warm. I didn't finish my cereal.

My mother introduced me to another kind of cereal later on. It was cereal made with leftover cornbread. The recipe follows.

Cornbread Cereal

Preparation time: 10 minutes
Cooking time: 20 minutes
Serving size: 6

Ingredients:

1 box Jiffy cornbread muffin mix
1 egg white
⅓ C. almond or cashew milk
1 Tbs. Olive oil
½ C. orange flavored dried cranberries (optional)
½ C. roasted unsalted sunflower seeds (optional)

Directions:

Use olive oil to coat a 9 1/2 X 11 baking dish. Follow directions on the cornbread muffin mix to make and bake cornbread. I use cornbread mix for convenience. To make scratch cornbread if you're feeling ambitious and not pressed for time, see the recipe below.

Serve:

Spoon about a 2-inch square corner of cornbread into a bowl and crumble. Add cranberries, sunflower seeds and milk. When the cornbread is loosened by the milk, the cereal is ready to eat.

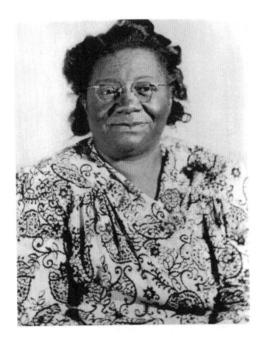

Annie Lee Ross my maternal grandmother

Scratch Cornbread

Preparation time: 10 minutes
Cooking time: 35 minutes
Serving size: 6

Ingredients:

1 C. Yellow Cornmeal
1 Tsp. Baking Soda
1 Tsp. Baking Powder
1½ C. Non-dairy milk
1 Non-dairy egg
3 Tbs. Non-dairy butter, melted
½ C. Unbleached white flour

Directions:

Preheat oven to 400 degrees. Oil a 9 X 11 baking dish or a 10" cast iron skillet. If you use the skillet, heat it in the oven before pouring the batter. In a large bowl whisk the egg and milk until well blended. Fold in the dry ingredients and melted butter to form a slightly lumpy batter. Pour the batter into the baking dish. If using the skillet, remove it from the oven to pour the batter; then return the batter-filled skillet to the oven. Bake the cornbread until the edges and top turn golden brown, about 30- 35 minutes. Let the cornbread cool about 10 minutes.

Serve:

Spoon about a 2-inch square corner of cornbread into a bowl and crumble. Add cranberries, sunflower seeds and milk. When the cornbread is loosened by the milk, the cereal is ready to eat.

Breakfast and Protein

Steak, bacon, sausage, and ham are meats typically associated with the first meal of the day and are especially lethal. Bacon, in its various forms—Canadian, turkey, pork—sausage, steak all have high fat, and high sodium content. In many cases the sodium is loads of nitrates. Why the need for breakfast meat? If our body needs protein, nutrients from vegetables or fruits and grains, doesn't that get satisfied with a breakfast of egg whites (protein), cantaloupe or grapefruit (fruit or vegetable nutrients), and toasted whole grain bread (grain)? Why do we need two proteins with our breakfast? It is just out of custom or habit that we have bacon AND eggs at breakfast. They are both protein sources, but we only need one. Sometimes food combinations or pairings we grew up with and for which we are accustomed, aren't good for us.

Cornbread is a food that is good for pairings with other foods. There was a song written about such pairings made popular in the late '40s and '50s. Thanks to my colleague Donzella Lee for bringing this song to my attention. Beans 'N' Cornbread made its way into the rhyming songs of children playing—especially little African American girls, I imagine jumping rope. The lyrics here illustrate how prevalent food pairing is to the American diet.

> Beans 'n' cornbread had a fight
> Beans knocked cornbread out of sight
> Cornbread said now that's alright
> Meet me on the corner tomorrow night
> I'll be ready tomorrow night
>
> Beans told cornbread you ain't straight
> You better wake up or I'll gas you gate
> Been in this pot since half past two
> Swelling and puffing and almost do
> I'll be ready tomorrow night
>
> Beans grabbed cornbread by the toe
> Beans said cornbread let me go
> Cornbread said I'll lay you low
> I'm gonna fight you, you so & so
> Meet on the corner tomorrow night

Beans hit cornbread on the head
Cornbread said I'm almost dead,
Beans told cornbread get up man
You know that we go hand-in-hand
We should hang out together like:
Like wieners and sauerkraut,
Like hot dogs and mustard
Like sisters and brothers,
Like chittlin's and potato salad,
Like strawberry & shortcake,
Like corn beef and cabbage,
Like liver & onions,
Like red beans & rice,
Like bagels & lox,
Like sour cream and biscuits,
Like bread & butter,
Like hot cakes & molasses
Beans told cornbread

Makes no difference what you think about me,
But makes a whole lot of difference what I think about you
That's what beans said to cornbread 'cause
Beans 'n' cornbread...they go hand-in-hand

Beans 'N' Cornbread (1949 – Louis Jordan & The Tympany Five)

I have made new discoveries of breakfast foods that go hand-in-hand and, while meatless, are full of protein as in the recipes that follow.

Egg White, Spinach and Mushroom Omelet

Preparation time: 0 minutes
Cooking time: 15 minutes
Serving size: 2

Ingredients:

1 C. Spinach, packaged
1 C. Crimini mushrooms, sliced
½ or equivalent of 2 Whites of eggs or packaged egg whites
   (Egg Beaters, Reddi-Egg, etc.)
½ Tsp. Olive oil
¼ Tsp. Black pepper, ground

Directions:

In an omelet pan or skillet, heat olive oil over medium heat. Add mushrooms and cook until tender. Add spinach. Cook the spinach for about 5 minutes or until leaves are bright green color and tender. Add egg whites and pepper. Cook until egg is firm. Fold into an omelet or stir for scrambled eggs.

Serve:

Plate with fresh fruit side dish—strawberries, cantaloupe, blueberries, etc.

Oatmeal: my opinion

I never liked oatmeal. I can't be sure, but I believe an early name for it was gruel. That name seems appropriate. The texture and consistency is vile. No matter in what style it's prepared or how you dress it up. To me it looks like something you've already eaten. I gagged every time I tried to eat it. It is reported to be an excellent food for combating most heart disease conditions, due to its high fiber content. Still I find it hard to keep down. It's a matter of preference. I have found other high fiber substitutes for those of us who can't stomach oatmeal. Granola is wonderful. It can be eaten as a hot or cold cereal with other than dairy milk.

Granola & Berries

Preparation time: 0 minutes
Cooking time: 0 minutes
Serving size: 10-12

Ingredients:

½ C. Dried oats, ground
½ C. Barley, ground
½ C. Brown Rice, ground
½ C. Almonds, shaved
½ C. Raisins, dried dates or cranberries

Directions:

This is a fantastic source of fiber. The ingredients can be found at most full service supermarkets, health food stores and health stores like GNC. If the oats, barley and rice are unground use your food processor to grind them. Mix all the ingredients together for granola. You may add your own ingredients like dried dates, cranberries, raisins etc. for added flavor.

For granola bars add applesauce enough to bind the mixture. Shape the mixture as you wish and refrigerate the bars until firm.

Quinoa, Nuts & Fresh Fruit

Preparation time: 5 minutes
Cooking time: 30 minutes
Serving size: 2-4

Ingredients:

1 C. White Quinoa
2 C. Almond milk
¼ C. Maple Syrup, pure
1 Tsp. Cinnamon
½ C. Raisins, dried dates or cranberries
1 Fuji Apple, diced

Directions:

In a quart saucepan, bring 2 cups of milk to a boil. Stir in 1 cup of white quinoa. Bring the quinoa to a boil, then reduce the flame, stir in the maple syrup, butter and allow the quinoa to simmer, covered until all the water is absorbed.

Spoon the hot quinoa into a bowl. Add the cinnamon, nuts, and apple to mix with the hot quinoa.

Serve:

Warm

APPETIZERS & SNACKS

From the age of 10 through about 14, I'd come home from school famished. I'd feel like I hadn't eaten in days when in fact, I'd had lunch at school probably a sandwich of some kind, chips and drink followed by a sticky bun. By 3:30 in the afternoon I was ready to eat again. Signs of a growing child I guess.

Both my aunt and uncle worked. When we arrived home, we were on our own. Being on our own after school would later be known as "latch key kids." We were left to our own devices and creativity to feed the afterschool hunger. We'd change from our school clothes into our "play" clothes and have at it in the kitchen. Each day the snack would be a little different.

One day something with peanut butter and jelly. Another day it was a mayonnaise (Miracle Whip) and sugar sandwich. Sometimes it would simply be bread and butter. Not a sandwich, just a single piece of bread with butter spread on it folded over. Those were the days. Shows how our tastes mature. Not only is a snack like that repulsive today, but just thinking about eating such stuff clogs my arteries.

Whatever the concoction I'd dream up, it was always ready to enjoy in time for viewing Dark Shadows with Barnabus Collins and company. What follows are healthier more appealing snacks.

Bean & Avocado Layered Crisp

Preparation time: 15 minutes
Cooking time: 45 minutes
Serving size: 8 crisps

Ingredients:

½ C. mashed white or navy beans
2 Tbs. minced garlic
4 C. vegetable broth
½ C. Roma tomatoes, diced
½ C. ripe olives, sliced
8-10 quartered multi-grained bread slices or sliced baguette, toasted

Directions:

Soak beans for a minimum of 8 hours. Place soaked beans in a 1- quart sauce pan with the garlic and vegetable broth. Bring the combination to a boil. Reduce the flame to medium-low and let the beans simmer until tender. Remove tender beans from heat. Place them in a mixing bowl and mash the beans with a fork or potato masher until all beans are mashed into a rough paste. Cut the avocado in half and scoop out the contents of the hull into another bowl, removing the pit. Mash the avocado until it forms a soft paste. Beginning with the beans, layer the ingredients avocado, tomatoes and olives one on another for each slice of toasted baguette or bread until all ingredients are used.

Serve:

Place the bean and avocado crisps on a dish to serve.

White Bean/Avocado Dip

Preparation time: 15 minutes
Cooking time: 45 minutes
Serving size: 6-8

Ingredients:

2 C. Dry white beans, soaked
4 C. Vegetable stock
2 Avocados
½ C. Pepperoncini juice
1 Tsp. Black pepper, ground
1 Tsp. Turmeric, ground
4 Garlic cloves, minced

Directions:

In a 2-quart sauce pan place the soaked white beans and add vegetable broth. On a high flame, bring the beans to a boil. Turn down the flame to low and simmer until beans are tender about 30 minutes. For added flavor, you could season the boiling beans with garlic and turmeric. Place the cooked beans in 9-quart food processor with half pepperoncini juice and mix. Cut and scoop out avocados placing them in the food processor, along with garlic, black pepper, and remaining pepperoncini juice. Combine the ingredients until smooth.

Serve:

Spoon the mixture into a bowl and add celery spears, broccoli, carrot sticks or chips of your choice on the side.

Nut Butter and Celery Sticks

Preparation time: 2 minutes
Cooking time: 0 minutes
Serving size: 4-6

Ingredients:

½ C. Nut butter (almond, cashew)
4 Celery Stalks

Directions:

For homemade nut butter, see the appendix. I offer almond and cashew as alternatives to peanuts for those of us allergic to peanuts. You can probably use any nut—Filberts or Brazil for instance. I feature my most favorite nuts. Slice celery stalks length-wise into strips. 4-stalks should yield 8 strips, 2 strips per stalk, then cut the stalks in half width-wise for 16 strips. To serve, place nut butter in a small serving dish for dipping celery. The nut butter can also be spread on the celery. Or, for serving to children under 5 years old, spread the butter on whole celery, then cut celery width-wise into bite-sized pieces for little fingers.

Garbanzo Bean, Avocado, Onion Sandwich

Preparation time: 15 minutes
Cooking time: 0 minutes
Serving size: 2

Ingredients:

½ C. Garbanzo Beans (soaked, cooked)
1 Avocado
½ Yellow onion, small sliced
4 Tbs. non-dairy butter
1 Tbs. Garlic, minced
1 Tsp. Horseradish
4 slices bread
½ Tsp. Black pepper, ground

Directions:

Mash tender cooked beans until they become a paste. It isn't necessary to mash them until they are smooth. Roughly mashed gives the paste a bit of texture. Stir garlic into the paste and add black pepper mixing thoroughly. Spread non-dairy butter over each slice of bread and toast. Spread the bean paste on the toasted bread. Spread horseradish over bean paste, then add onion slices and top with avocado. Place the remaining toast on top of the avocado to complete the sandwich.

Serve:

Cut the sandwich in half at a diagonal and serve with green pea crisps or kale chips.

The Jalopy and Abbot's Frozen Custard

It was a beet red 1950 Plymouth roadster convertible. Imagine that. It was the summer of 1963 or so, my uncle came home all excited about this car he found. The other car must have given out. We were bus dependent for a time. He found a deal on this 2-door Plymouth that would help the family be mobile again. My uncle was pretty thrifty to say the very least, and always looking for an opportunity to pay as little as possible for goods and services. This must've been a good deal.

For car enthusiasts, I know the Plymouth is considered a classic. Uncle wasn't a car enthusiast. He wasn't a mechanic. He didn't buy the car to restore it to its original glory. Buying the car was purely utilitarian. We needed transportation. He urged us to come see it and take a test drive. After all, it was a convertible.

We went down to the parking lot to see this fabulous car he was raving about. Oh my goodness. The beet red paint on the car had dulled. It had a mat finish by circumstance not by design. The convertible top had tears in it. The interior was dark with dreary torn upholstery covering the seats. Floor boards were missing. You could see the ground from inside the car. We could use our feet to stop the car if we had to—like the Flintstone cartoon.

My uncle suggested we take a drive to the beach for Abbott's frozen custard to test ride the car. I was against it. Not me, you all go ahead. I was about 11 or 12 years old at the time. I was not among the cool kids as it was and being seen in this piece of junk wasn't going to help my reputation. At that age, reputation was important. I'll pass. Somehow, I got talked into going. So I piled into the backseat with the 4 other kids—my two sisters Diane and Barbara, cousins Joan and Anita. In a group of kids, no one would recognize me. So off we went.

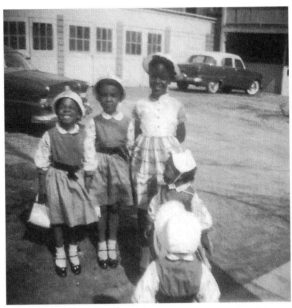

From right: Me, Diane, Joan, Barbara is standing in front of me.
Anita has her back to the camera. Dressed for Easter Sunday.

As we drove down the street, we could see the pavement passing under us. Part of the convertible top loose from the frame was flapping in the wind. How embarrassing. Not cool. One of the kids pointed out the flapping top. Hearing that and unfazed, uncle decided to lower the top. The lower the convertible top, the further down the seat I slid. I couldn't be seen in this beat up mess. This is way before the time seat belts became mandatory. When we were out of our neighborhood, I felt more comfortable about being seen. No one knows me here, and I don't ever have to again face anyone who sees me. I sat up straight and joined the other kids in waving at people we passed. The hot summer air felt light and cool on my face and got cooler the closer we came to the beach. This isn't so bad. All we needed was the radio. It didn't work, of course. If it did, it might've drowned out the loud, harsh engine sound. But we got used to it by the time we reached our destination.

We pulled into a parking space in front of Abbott's. People were staring. It isn't every day you see a car full of young Black kids in the backseat of a convertible in 1963. We stayed in the car while uncle ordered the treat. We had our choice of vanilla, chocolate, or strawberry. I got vanilla. It was heavenly. After the frozen custard, being seen in the dilapidated car didn't matter so much anymore.

Frozen custard hasn't been available outside of Rochester until recently. Fruit smoothies have been my answer to the absent frozen custard. Smoothies are just as rich and creamy as the custard. Using seasonal fruit provides flavor variety. I find that bananas combined with any other fruit add depth to the taste and balance to the texture. We are lucky in California to have such a myriad of fruit available at a much longer time than other regions of the continent. What follows are a few smoothie recipes that will stir your creativity.

Strawberry, Banana Smoothie

Preparation time: 10 minutes
Cooking time: 0 minutes
Serving size: 2, 8-oz glasses

Ingredients:

2 Bananas, frozen
½ C. Strawberries, frozen
2 C. Almond milk

Directions:

Add milk, banana and strawberries to a blender. Blend on smoothie or high speed until all ingredients are smoothly blended.

Serve:

Pour contents of the blender into a tall 8-oz glass.

Malik's Mixed Fruit Smoothie

Preparation time: 10 minutes
Cooking time: 0 minutes
Serving size: 2, 8-oz glasses

Ingredients:

½ C. Banana
½ C. Mixed fruit – blue berries, strawberries, pineapple
1 C. Ice
1 C. Spinach
1 C. milk or apple juice
½ C. Chia seeds

Directions:

Add all ingredients beginning with the fruit to a blender. Blend on smoothie or high speed until all ingredients are smoothly blended.

Serve:

Pour contents of the blender into an 8-oz. glass.

Stuffed Mushrooms

Preparation time: 30 minutes
Cooking time: 45 minutes
Serving size: 32-48 mushrooms

Ingredients:

3 pt. White or button mushrooms
¼ C. Italian salad dressing

Directions:

Clean and blot dry mushrooms. Remove the mushroom stems and center with a knife or spoon and set aside. [These pieces can be refrigerated for use in sauces, soups, etc.].

Heat oven to 375 degrees; follow the recipe for oyster dressing herein. Coat mushroom caps with Italian salad dressing. Use the oyster dressing mixture to stuff inside the mushroom caps. Place the stuffed mushrooms in a shallow baking dish. Place the dish in the oven and cook for 45 minutes or until mushroom caps are fork tender.

Locked In

I was about 7 on this particular occasion when my mother was cleaning the refrigerator after breakfast. It was a new refrigerator not an icebox. After all this was the late 1950s. Maybe 1958.

Unlike the icebox, the refrigerator stood tall and upright. It was powered by electricity and had a freezer compartment within it that held trays to freeze water. My mother turned off the refrigerator to clean it so that it was no longer generating coolness. In addition to taking out all the food stored there to give it a thorough cleaning she removed shelves, drawers and anything that was removable to clean every nook and cranny. The phone rang and mother left the refrigerator to answer the call. There stood an empty refrigerator with the door open wide, light shining bright. The empty cavity was so inviting. It called to me. Besides, my 7 year old curiosity wanted to know if the refrigerator light remained on once the door closed. I climbed in.

Fitting snugly with my feet tucked under me. I closed the door and everything went dark. My question was answered. I now knew that the light went out when the door closed. Mother still on the phone hadn't noticed my climb into the empty refrigerator. She talked for several minutes. My curiosity satisfied, I wanted out. Well there's no way to open the door from the inside. Mother still into her phone conversation didn't return to finish the cleaning job right away. From inside I began to bang on the door. My sister Diane finally heard me and told mother I was inside the refrigerator. Mother ended her call and rushed to the refrigerator to get me out. I expected to get a spanking, but didn't. She just yelled at me, telling me never to do that again. You could suffocate, she said. She peppered me with suppositions—suppose Diane didn't hear you; suppose, I didn't return to finish cleaning the refrigerator right away; suppose, suppose, suppose. Looking back, I think she was more frightened than I was.

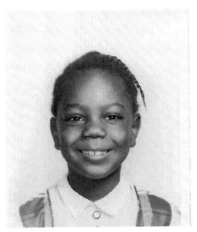

Me at about the age I decided to crawl into the empty refrigerator.

In those days, I remember eating plenty of soups for lunch. Tomato, alphabet, and chicken noodle soups were my favorite. We'd have saltine crackers with it. Knowing what I know now, that's a lot of sodium. Sodium in the canned soup and the crackers. I certainly can't eat what I use to, but discovered this Lentil and other soup recipes that are low sodium yet full of flavor.

SOUPS & STEWS

When the weather turns cold in fall your clothing changes to sweaters and socks and at the end of the day you feel like covering up with a throw blanket on the couch to read a good book, watch great television or snuggle with someone special. It's the time of year my meals tend towards dishes that warm your insides. I also seek dishes that have some staying power like soups and stews. Living in Los Angeles, we don't have distinctive seasons, but it does get cooler in the fall. We don't need the heavy meals typically associated with mid-westerners or those of you who live in the northeast who must fortify yourselves against the elements. However, we do find single-pot and slow cooked meals provide the warmth and comfort we seek for a cold fall or winter night. Wherever you call home when the weather turns cold, you'll find the following dishes satisfying especially when paired with a generous hunk of warmed crusty bread spread with garlic butter. Garlic butter is mentioned in several recipes. I make my own. You'll find a "how to" in the appendix.

Lentil Soup with Spinach

Preparation time: 15 minutes
Cooking time: 60 minutes
Serving size: 6 Bowls

Ingredients:

2 C. Dry lentil beans, soaked
4 Garlic cloves, minced
½ Tsp. Olive oil
1 Tsp. Turmeric
2 C. Spinach
1 Yellow onion (optional), sliced; *1 large leek could be used either in combination or as an onion replacement.*
6 C. Vegetable broth, organic, low-sodium

Directions:

In a sauce pan, heat oil over low flame. Add garlic and stir until heated and fragrant. If you use onion, add it at this time and cook until caramelized. The caramelized onion brings a hint of sweetness to the soup that balances the beans' smoky, savory flavor and the bitterness of the spinach to be added towards the end of cooking. If leeks are used, they should be sliced and cooked as you would the onion. Pour in vegetable broth followed by the soaked lentil beans. Increase the flame to high until the broth boils. When the pan contents begin to boil, turn down the flame and allow the beans to simmer until tender. Add spinach to the last 5 minutes of cooking to give the soup color interest. The spinach should be tender and bright green.

Serve:

Place in soup bowl with a piece of crusty bread on the side (the bread is optional, of course).

These single-pot, slow-cooked meals usually start by sautéing mirepoix. Chefs are familiar with this word and method. It's a French word pronounced meer-pwah. Mirepoix is a combination of chopped onions, celery, and carrots used in soups, stews and stocks for flavor and richness. Mirepoix begins the recipes that follow. Although I don't name it, you'll find that method as part of the cooking directions throughout the book.

Vegetable Soup

Preparation time: 30 minutes
Cooking time: 90 minutes
Serving size: 6-8 Bowls

Ingredients:

2 C. Dry Navy beans, soaked
4 Garlic cloves, minced
2 Yellow onions, medium-sized, diced
4 Carrots, sliced into medallions
4 Celery stalks with leaves, sliced
2 White potatoes, diced in large
 pieces
½ Tbs. Olive oil

1 Tsp. Turmeric
4 Bay leaves
1 Tbs. Cumin
1 Tbs. Cardamom
½ Tbs. Coriander
3 C. Vegetable broth, organic, low-
 sodium
3 C. Water

Directions:

In a 10-quart Dutch oven or pan, heat oil over low flame. Add onions, carrots, celery, and garlic. Heat them until the onions become translucent the other vegetables are fragrant. Add vegetable broth and stir. Increase the flame to medium.

When the broth begins to bubble, add the potatoes and spices including bay leaves. Stir the ingredients. Add water to the pot. When the pan contents begin to boil, turn down the flame and allow the beans to simmer until tender.

Serve:

Place in soup bowl with a piece of crusty bread on the side (the bread is optional, of course).

The only difference between soups and stews is the amount of pot liquor it's cooked in. This next stew recipe is hearty enough to satisfy all manner of appetites.

Root Vegetable Stew

Preparation time: 30 minutes
Cooking time: 90 minutes
Serving size: 8 Bowls

Ingredients:

2 C. Dry Pinto beans, soaked
[or the bean of your choice]
5 Tbs. Garlic, minced
[heaping tablespoons]
2 Yellow onions, large, quartered
4 Carrots, rainbow, medallion
sliced
4 Celery stalks with leaves, sliced
2 White potatoes, diced in large
pieces
2 Parsnips, medallion sliced
1 Fennel bulb, sliced
¼ lbs. Collard greens, fresh

8 oz. Mushrooms, baby bellas
½ Tbs. Olive oil
1 Tsp. Turmeric
4 Bay leaves
1 Tbs. Cumin
1 Tbs. Cardamom
½ Tbs. Coriander
½ Tbs. Nutmeg
2 Tbs. Pepper, ground peppercorn
6 C. Vegetable broth, organic,
low-sodium
2 C. Water

Directions:

In a 10-quart Dutch oven or pan, heat oil over low flame. Add onions, carrots, celery, and garlic. Heat them until the onions become translucent and the other vegetables are fragrant. Add vegetable broth and stir. Increase the flame to medium. When the broth begins to bubble, add the remaining root vegetables—potatoes, parsnip, fennel, mushrooms and all spices, except the nutmeg. Place the bay leaves in the pot. Allow the ingredients to simmer on a medium to low flame.

Cooked fennel brightens the stew with a bit of sweetness along with the carrots to counter the savory from the other ingredients as it simmers. Stir the ingredients occasionally. Add water to the pot but not too much. Fennel, onion to an extent, collards and mushrooms generate their own flavor enhancing liquid—pot liquor.

While the root vegetables simmer, wash the collard greens and remove the leaves from the large thick stem. Cut them cross-wise into strips and add them to the pot followed by the nutmeg. Nutmeg remember takes away the bitter taste of the dark greens. Stir in the drained, soaked beans. Increase the flame to high until the liquid boils. When the pot begins to boil, turn down the flame and allow the stew to simmer until the beans and greens are tender about 90 minutes.

Serve:

Place the stew in deep bowl along with a piece of crusty bread on the side (the bread is optional, of course).

SALADS

Cucumber Radish Onion Salad

Preparation time: 10 minutes
Cooking time: 0 minutes
Serving size: 4

Ingredients:

1 Cucumber
4 Radishes, medium-size
1 Yellow onion
1 Tbs. Fennel seeds

Dressing
3 Tbs. Apple cider vinegar
2 Tsp. Agave
1 Tsp. Extra Virgin Olive Oil

Directions:

Scrub clean the cucumber and radishes. Peel the "cuke" to show some of the green. Into a dish, thinly slice the cucumber and radishes into medallions. Remove the onion hull and cut the onion in half length-wise. With the flat side down on the cutting board, thinly slice the onion across its width. Add the onion to the bowl of cucumbers and radishes. Sprinkle in fennel seeds. Using your hands toss the ingredients together breaking up the onion into individual pieces and set it aside.

To make the dressing, mix together apple cider vinegar, agave and olive oil until the ingredients are blended. Drizzle the dressing over the salad and serve.

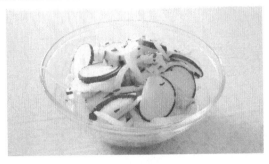

Tomato, Avocado, Red Onion Salad

Preparation time: 20 minutes
Cooking time: 0 minutes
Serving size: 6

Ingredients:

4 Tomatoes (Roma or hot house), diced
2 Avocados, diced
½ Red Onion, diced
½ C. Cooked Shrimp (optional)
3 Tbs. Balsamic Vinaigrette dressing

Directions:

In a medium bowl, mix ingredients together. Drizzle dressing over ingredients. Refrigerate for a minimum of 3 hours to allow flavors to mingle.

Serve:

Plate over a bed of lettuce or on its own.

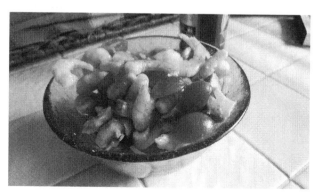

Not Your Grandma's Potato Salad

Preparation time: 30 minutes
Cooking time: 10-20 minutes
Serving size: 6

Ingredients:

5 – 6 Medium-size potatoes, cut
   chunky
2 C. Vegetable broth
8 oz. Peas
¼ Onion, grated
4 Radishes, quartered
4 Granny Smith Apples, peeled &
   shoe stringed
½ Lemon

4 oz. Capers
2 Tbs. Chives
2 Tbs. Dill

Dressing
4 Tbs. Apple cider vinegar
¼ C. Dijon mustard
2 Tbs. Honey
1 Tbs. Olive Oil
¼ Tsp. Black pepper, coarse

Directions:

Place potatoes (skin on) in medium sauce pan and add vegetable broth. Bring the potatoes to a boil and reduce flame to continue boiling until just tender.

While the potatoes are cooking, clean and remove stems and roots from the radishes. Cut them into quarters and set aside. Peel the apples using a vegetable peeler. Core them and cut into shoestring shape. Squeeze lemon juice on the cut apples to prevent discoloration and set them aside. Chop up the dill and chives.

When the potatoes are tender remove them from the heat and drain the vegetable broth from the potatoes placing them in a large mixing bowl. Set aside remaining vegetable broth for future use. While the potatoes are cooling make the salad dressing.

Salad Dressing

Whisk the mustard and vinegar together in a small mixing bowl until combined. Pour in the honey tasting as you go and continue to whisk until there's a blend of sweet and tangy. Fold in remaining ingredients until well blended.

Add to the mixing bowl of potatoes all of the salad ingredients from above, the peas, onion, apple, radishes, capers, dill and chives. Mix them together until they are well blended. Fold in the dressing until all ingredients are coated. Refrigerate the potato salad until chilled and Serve: on a lettuce leaf.

ENTREES & SIDE DISHES

Whenever we had greens—mustard, turnip, dandelion or collard— as a side dish with the meal, they were usually boiled with pork for flavor. It would take up to three hours to cook them until they were "tender." Greens were most often part of the Sunday menu when there was more cooking time. Actually, cooking them in that way for that length of time reduces the nutrients the greens provide. When properly cooked, they are a rich source of iron, fiber, and combats cancer.

This next recipe is an example of a hearty, tasty meal with greens that takes only 30 minutes.

Beans 'n' Greens

Preparation time: 5 minutes
Cooking time: 30 minutes
Serving size: 4

Ingredients:

1 lb. Collard or mixed country
  greens (mustard, turnip, kale)
4 Garlic cloves (or more if you like)
2 Tbs. Olive oil

1 C. Vegetable broth
1 Tsp. Red pepper, crushed
1 Tsp. Nutmeg, powdered
1 C. Navy or white beans, cooked

Directions:

Heat olive oil in a sauce pan or sauté pan over medium to low flame. Add garlic until their aroma is released. Add greens. Coat greens with oil and garlic. Add vegetable broth and cook until nearly tender. Add crushed pepper and nutmeg and stir. A little known fact, nutmeg helps to diminish the bitterness of the collards or any bitter green. I learned that it's used in plenty of Mediterranean dishes. Add vegetable broth as needed to the greens to allow them to simmer and the flavors to mingle until greens are tender. Stir in beans until they are heated. Remove from heat and serve.

Serve:

Plate the greens with white beans and let stand for 1 minute before dining.

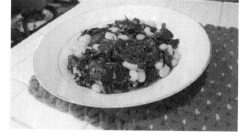

Tamales

Once a year my aunt would make beef tamales from scratch. The beef was purchased from a butcher. My aunt ground the beef. She used cornmeal to make the filling. She'd stuff the filling into corn husks she collected throughout the year and dried. She'd steam the tamales in big roasting pans. It is such a massive project that once a year was all she could devote to it. It wasn't necessarily at holiday time as in the tradition of Latin Americans. She made them when the mood hit her.

When I moved to the west coast, I learned my aunt's recipe is authentic. They tasted as good, as fresh, as tamales made by people of Spanish descent. Where she learned it I'll never know. She was African-American born and raised in Ohio. She never shared the recipe before her death. You won't find a vegetarian version among the recipes in this book. I share this story here to give a sense of the foods I was exposed to growing up.

While I don't have a plant-based substitute for my aunt's tamales, I do have a recipe that is as tasty as Aunt Ida's tamales and very much a production. In homage to Wednesday and spaghetti night, I offer a plant-based lasagna recipe.

Lasagna

Preparation time: 2 hours
Cooking time: 1 hour
Serving size: 8

Ingredients:

1 Eggplant, sliced length-wise
2 Zucchini (optional)
2 C. Kidney beans, cooked and ground
½ Cauliflower florets, minced
1 lbs Tomato sauce

4 Tbs. Oregano, dried ground
4 Tbs. Basil, dried ground or 4 oz. fresh
4 Tbs. Olive oil
1 Bell pepper, diced
1 Brown Onion, diced

Directions:

It might be best to approach this recipe in 3 stages. The first stage is the vegetable preparation. The cooked kidney beans need to be put through a food processor to grind them. Place the ground kidney beans in a container for later. Cut the cauliflower florets off the stem. Place them in a food processor to chop them until they look like course, grainy cheese. Put them aside. Slice the eggplant length-wise. They can be put aside. Slice the zucchini into medallions.

The second stage is the sauce preparation. In a deep pot, heat the olive oil over a medium flame. Once the oil is heated place onion in the pan and heat until translucent. Add bell pepper and cook until tender. To the onion and bell pepper add the tomato sauce. Stir in basil and oregano. Increase the flame to high until the sauce bubbles. Reduce the flame and simmer for 90 minutes.

The third stage is assembling the ingredients to make the lasagna. In a 9 1/2 " X 11" baking dish layer the ingredients in the following order until all the ingredients are used: Eggplant, ground kidney beans, zucchini, tomato sauce, and cauliflower. The final layer should end with cauliflower. Place the dish in a 350 degree oven and bake until the sauce bubbles and the cauliflower is browned. Depending on the oven, the baking time could be 45-60 minutes.

Serve:

Remove the baking dish from the oven and let stand for 15 minutes. Cut the lasagna into squares and serve warm.

This is fairly labor intense, but worth it for the flavor. This sizeable dish is good for dinner parties or can provide several meals in the course of a week. Over time the flavors of the ingredients blend and add to the taste.

As a substitute for meat-centered Sunday meals and perhaps Monday leftovers, below are more hearty plant-based recipes.

White Quinoa, Fennel & Mushrooms

Preparation time: 20 minutes
Cooking time: 30 minutes
Serving size: 4 meals

Ingredients:

1 C. White quinoa, cooked
1 Onion, yellow
2 Fennel bulbs
1 C. Crimini mushrooms
3 Anchovy fillets

1 Tbs. Olive Oil, Extra Virgin
1 C. Vegetable Broth
½ C. Green onion
½ Tsp Curry

Directions:

Quinoa, pronounced Keen-wha, is a grain consisting of nearly pure protein. It's cooked like rice. Follow directions on the package but instead of water use vegetable broth for added flavor. In a sauce pan cook a cup of quinoa in 2 cups of vegetable broth with curry and green onion added. Bring it to a boil, then simmer for 20 minutes or until all the liquid is absorbed. Set the quinoa aside to cool.

In a sauté pan add olive oil and heat under medium flame until hot. Add onion to caramelize*. Once the onion is caramelized, set it aside in a dish. Add another tablespoon of olive oil and a tablespoon of non-dairy butter to the sauté pan. When it is heated, add the fennel. Cook until the fennel is al dente. Set the fennel aside in a separate dish. Add a 1/2 tablespoon of oil to the same pan. When the oil is heated, add mushrooms and cook in a covered pan until the mushrooms make a juice and are brown on both sides. To the mushrooms return the caramelized onion and fennel to the pan.

Place 3 strips of anchovies in the pan with the vegetables. Stir until the anchovies are integrated into the vegetables. Add vegetable broth and simmer for 5 minutes with the lid off. Turn off the flame. The vegetables are ready to serve with the quinoa.

For most of the recipes in this book, you are encouraged to use your instincts and be inspired by your own palate when it comes to taste and ingredient amounts. In time, one learns a few short cuts in a cooking process or technique. For this recipe, however, using short cuts will give a different flavor experience.

Serve:

To plate the dish, spoon two heaping serving spoons of quinoa onto a plate. Spoon the vegetables over the quinoa with a little of the juice and enjoy.

* Caramelized is a sauté cooking technique that essentially browns the onion bringing out a sweet flavor.

On Sodium

Those of us with hypertension or high blood pressure are warned by our doctors to stay far away from sodium or salt. Sodium is not our friend. Sodium chloride is the chemical name for salt. (Prevention, 2013) I use the terms interchangeably. These days, there are different kinds of salt with different textures used to flavor or texturize food. Sea salt, Himalayan, kosher, etc. Some claim to provide better or additional nutrients than regular iodized table salt. No matter what name or texture, too much sodium elevates blood pressure by causing our blood vessels to constrict or contract. (Prevention, 2013)

High amounts of sodium are found in most processed foods to extend their shelf life. As much as possible with a few exceptions, I recommend cooking with fresh ingredients rather than processed foods. Take a look at food labels. I never add sodium/salt to my food. You won't find salt/sodium in any of the recipes herein. Herbs, spices and other ingredients replace sodium. After a while you won't miss it. When you have meals away from home, you'll know immediately when sodium has been added. I learned that certain foods naturally contain sodium like celery, tomatoes and spinach.

Sodium was originally used to preserve foods before refrigeration. With refrigeration, the need for salt as a preservative has diminished. (MacGregor, 2007, pp. 18-54) Although sodium is no longer necessary to preserve food, its content remains high in processed foods. The rationale for the continued use is that sodium continues to reduce pathogens and organisms that spoil some processed food products and reduce their shelf life. (JE Henney, 2010) In some foods salt improves food texture. (JE Henney, 2010)

Taste and flavors connected to sodium use historically is an expectation. However, it isn't necessary to add sodium to freshly cooked food.

This will seem like a contradiction...

While I encourage fresh, wholesome unprocessed foods, there are times when I use canned, bottled, boxed or frozen foods for convenience. This next recipe is an example. Chili requires tomato sauce. If you can take the time to make tomato sauce and stewed tomatoes, that is preferable. Instructions on how to make tomato sauce are in this book's appendix. Rather than make my own tomato sauce or stewed tomatoes, I buy the canned versions. Using canned beans along with canned tomato sauce and stewed tomatoes multiplies the chili's sodium content. To avoid that, when I use canned tomato sauce I use dried beans.

Chili

Preparation time: 15 minutes
Cooking time: 2 hours 30 minutes
Serving size: 16 cups

Ingredients:

Dry beans, soaked
1 C. White Navy or Great
    Northern
1 C. Red Kidney
1 C. Black
½ C. Corn (organic, if at all)
2-16 oz. cans Tomato Sauce
2-8 oz. cans Stewed Tomatoes

1 Onion, yellow or brown - diced
1 C. Green onion - sliced
1 Bell/Green pepper - diced
2 Tbs. Chili powder or to taste
1 Tbs. Turmeric
2 Bay leaves
½ C. Vegetable broth
1 Tbs. Olive oil

Directions:

Coat a 10-quart Dutch oven with olive oil. When olive oil is heated, add onion and bell pepper. Turn the flame to medium, cook until onion is translucent and the bell pepper is fragrant. Add tomato sauce and stewed tomatoes. Turn the flame to high. Drain the soaked beans and add them along with the bay leaves to the sauce mixture. When the mixture begins to boil, turn the flame down low and add chili powder, turmeric and stir. Simmer until all beans are tender about 90 minutes. Add corn and simmer another 30 minutes.

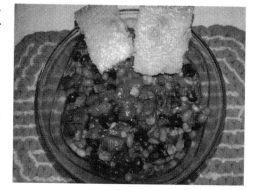

Serve:

In a bowl with cornbread. Ladle chili into a bowl. Add green onion to garnish and cornbread on the side.

The Van Voorhris Family

There must have been about 10 kids that lived in the house two doors down from us on St. Claire Street. We lived in a duplex on the corner of St. Claire and Tremont Streets at that time. The Van Voorhris' were the only remaining white family for blocks. Anita was about a year older than me. I was in second grade, which means I must have been 7 years old. My mother was alive then. Anita and her younger brother, Henry used to come over to play with me and my sister Diane. I remember thinking how the name Henry seemed like an adult name for such a little boy. Henry and Diane must have been about the same age—5 years old.

During the summer, when we were on school break, Anita would be up before dawn, it seemed, and come to my house, stand outside and yell my name in three melodic syllables…Gwen—doe-lyn-n-n. Besides the birds chirping, Anita's voice was all you could hear at that time of morning. Her voice was loud enough for the entire block to hear. I don't know why she felt the need to do that. I hadn't gotten out of bed yet let alone had breakfast. And there she was ready to play. We'd play hopscotch, jacks or ride our bikes up and down the street. Our end of Tremont Street was a dead end. There was hardly any traffic. On occasion, we'd get pretty creative in our play. I remember a time, when we decided to put on a play/musical.

We made a stage out of cardboard boxes. We used hair brushes for microphones. Old hand me down clothes became our costumes. I don't remember what the play/musical was about, but I do know it was an original. Anita recruited her sisters and Henry to play parts. We created the story, improvised the dialogue, and had rehearsal in preparation for the play's debut. It took us all day.

When we thought we were ready to perform, we went about recruiting an audience. Anita grabbed the rest of her sisters and brothers, I reached out to the Bannisters across the street. Michael Bannister was about our age but at the time didn't want anything to do with us. His brother and sister were much older and of course just dismissed us. With all our recruiting we couldn't get enough people together at one time to perform. After all that hard work/play. The play/musical never debuted. We were very disappointed.

We worked on the play until we got hungry. We stopped to eat lunch—lunch was either peanut butter and jelly sandwiches, grilled cheese sandwiches or pork 'n' beans and hot dogs. We probably ate at each other's houses at least once. I think we both found that although we came from different backgrounds, what we ate wasn't all that different. Today, as adults our lunches would consist of recipes like the following.

Cabbage Wrap

Preparation time: 60 minutes
Cooking time: 60 minutes
Serving size: 6-8

Ingredients:

6-8 Cabbage leaves
9 C. Garbanzo beans, dried, and
  soaked
¼ C. Vegetable broth
1 Tbs. Olive oil
1 Garlic head
½ Onion, yellow, minced
4 stalks Green onion
2 stalks Celery, finely chopped
½ C. Crimini mushrooms, diced

¼ C. Bread crumbs (finely
  crumbled)
3 Tbs. Garlic Butter
¼ Tbs. Cardamom (Curry,
  optional)
2 Tbs. crushed red peppers
2 Tbs. Mint, finely chopped
1 Tsp. black pepper, ground
1 Tsp. cumin
¼ Tsp. coriander

Directions:

Soak garbanzo beans overnight. Drain them and place soaked garbanzo beans in food processor. Pulse the processor to make beans into a lumpy paste.

Using a 10" sauté pan, pour in enough olive oil to coat the bottom. While the pan is heating, slice the celery, and green onions. Place the celery, green onion, and mushrooms in the heated sauté pan and cook covered until the mushrooms are golden and juice is created. Mushrooms do create their own savory pot liquor that is delicious in most recipes.

Add garlic, celery, onions, mushrooms with the pot liquor and mint to the bean mixture. Stir in bread crumbs to act as a binder. Thoroughly blend the ingredients until they are all incorporated into the bean paste. With a grater, mince the yellow onion over the blended mix and stir. Add cardamom, crushed red pepper, cumin, coriander black pepper to taste. Once the seasonings have been completely folded into the mix, set it aside to let the flavors mingle while you prepare the baking dish. Those flavor combinations will make your mouth water. This tantalizing bean paste is the cabbage leaf filling.

Meanwhile, in a 10" sauté pan place enough vegetable broth to cover the bottom. Heat the broth until small bubbles begin to form. Place individual cabbage leaves in the heated broth until the leaf becomes pliable. Once the leaf is flexible remove it from the pan immediately and set them aside.

In a shallow 9" X 11" baking dish, rub a thin layer of garlic butter on the bottom and sides. Pour the remaining vegetable broth in the dish. The dish is now ready for the cabbage wraps.

To make the wraps, spread open the softened cabbage leaf. Spoon about 2 tablespoons of the bean filling onto the opened leaf. Wrap the leaf around the filling and fold the ends under. Place the filled cabbage leaf in the baking dish and repeat the process placing the wraps side-by-side until all the leaves and filling are used. Spread remaining garlic butter over the cabbage wraps and place the baking dish into a 350 degree oven. The garlic butter melts over the cabbage wrap and will bubble in the bottom of the dish.

Bake for about 30 minutes or until a portion of the cabbage leaves turn golden. Use a spatula to place on dish to serve.

Parsnips, Turnips, Beets, Leeks with Red Quinoa

Preparation time: 30 minutes
Cooking time: 60 minutes
Serving size: 4

Ingredients:

1 Parsnip, without greens
1 Turnip, without greens
½ lbs Turnip greens
2 Beets, with greens
½ lbs Beet greens

1 Leek, sliced medallions
2 Tbs. Olive oil
6 Garlic cloves, minced
2½ C. Vegetable broth
1 C. Red Quinoa

Directions:

Heat oven to 350 degrees; clean vegetables with vegetable brush to remove all dirt. Coat parsnips, turnips and beets with a teaspoon of olive oil; place root vegetables in a shallow baking dish with water. Bake until fork tender about 60 minutes.

While the root vegetables are baking, follow directions for cooking quinoa on the package. Replace water with 2 cups of vegetable broth. Stir in garlic and simmer until all water is absorbed and set aside.

Sauté leeks and vegetable greens in 1 tablespoon olive oil until leeks are translucent, greens are tender and aroma is released.

Serve:

Plate the quinoa. Add root vegetables, greens and leeks on top or alongside the quinoa.

Zucchini, Garbanzo Beans, Yellow Onion

Preparation time: 15 minutes
Cooking time: 25 minutes
Serving size: 2

Ingredients:

2 Zucchini, sliced into spears
1 Yellow Onion
1 C. Crimini mushrooms
4 Tbs. Sesame ginger vinaigrette

1 C. Vegetable broth
2 Tbs. Olive oil, extra virgin
1 C. Garbanzo beans

Directions:

Soak garbanzo beans in water for at least 6 hours. Drain the beans and place them in a sauce pan. Cover the beans with vegetable broth and boil until tender. Set the beans aside.

Marinate zucchini spears in vinaigrette for at least 1-hour. Slice onion width-wise. Heat oil in a sauté pan. Place onion in oil and sauté until translucent. Add zucchini spears along with vinaigrette and sauté until zucchini is al dente. Stir vegetables together in vinaigrette sauce and add mushrooms and remaining vegetable broth. When the zucchini and mushrooms are tender add the cooked beans to heat and serve.

Food Fight: Genetically Modified Organisms (GMO)

A raging debate is taking place as of this writing over the controversial issue of genetically modified organisms. Because this discourse has such profound implications for plant-based cooking and indeed generally for those of us who eat food in America, I thought some discussion on the matter should be included here. By the way, Europe already has restrictions on GMO foods.

The conversation is on the question of whether or not our food should be labeled to indicate GMO food products. I strongly believe our food should be GMO or non-GMO labeled just as we now have labels that inform us of sodium content, calorie count, nutrients and ingredients to help us determine whether or not to purchase and consume the product.

Genetically Modified Organisms (GMOs) have molecular structure altered or genetically engineered DNA to create a new organism that does not naturally occur or occur through traditional crossbreeding. (WHO, 2015)

Common GMO food products we know of include corn, soy, canola, commercially produced varieties of sugar beets, squash, and Hawaiian papaya. Proponents assert that GMO foods are safe and more nutritious; they benefit the environment; reduce use of pesticides; increase crop yield; are an extension of natural breeding and have no difference in risk than naturally bred crops. (Project, 2015)

GMO opponents claim that GMO crops can be toxic, allergenic or less nutritious than their natural counterparts; they can disrupt the ecosystem, damage vulnerable wild plant and animal populations and harm biodiversity; increase chemical inputs long term; once released harmful GMOs cannot be recalled from the environment. (Project, 2015)

As of this writing, the controversy has expanded to salmon. There's debate over genetically modified salmon to enhance the diminishing population of wild salmon. GMO opponents have coined the term franken-fish warning it will soon be showing up in some of the finest restaurants if it hasn't already.

What I know for certain is that when I eat non-organic corn, I have an allergic reaction—nasal congestion, watery eyes, running nose, sneezing. This reaction also happens when I eat products made from corn—like chips, relish, etc.

If there is no risk difference than naturally bred crops, and GMO foods are safe as the proponents claim, why not label? GMO labeling will help us make informed decisions about what we put into our bodies. It gives us a choice. Without the label, we have no choice. Those who oppose GMO labeling act as if we are incapable of making our own decisions. Project and WHO (World Health Organization) referenced above are two sources to begin your further exploration into this important issue.

From the Land to the Table

Through my work with dieticians as an adult, I learned about the evolution of food preparation in African American households. Because most of us are descended from families that worked on a farm or at the very least raised their own food, this might be true for your family too. Food—meats and some vegetables —were usually fried because it is the most expedient cooking method. After working the farm or raising your own food from sun rise to sunset, meals had to be prepared fast to feed hungry workers before bedtime, which in some cases meant sunset. Although we migrated off the farms and into urban settings and factory jobs, these farm practices of fast cooking persisted on the whole at least into the 1950s when convenience meals like frozen foods and T.V. dinners were introduced. My grandparents were not farmers, but lived in a small rural town and depended on the land for their food.

Come 'n' Get It!

My grandfather had only 1 leg. His leg was missing from just above the knee down. He was my grandmother's second husband and mother's stepfather. At the time I didn't know how he lost his leg. Later on, I learned it was lost to diabetes. He didn't use crutches or a wheel chair; he got around using a 3-legged stool. He'd lean his weight on the stool and use his remaining leg to move from one place to another. It was a remarkable sight to watch him with his one leg and a stool.

Grandpa became so adept at moving that way, he was able to "run" after chickens. On a visit to their house one time, I watched him move fast enough to catch a chicken he eyed for dinner. The bird fled for its life, wings flapping, squawking and scurrying as fast as it could. Once caught Grandpa wrung its neck, placed the still moving chicken in a pan, covering it with a lid until movement stopped. Next thing I knew, the chicken was on the dinner table. Knowing that the bird for dinner was what Grandpa caught and killed, I wouldn't eat it.

Looking back, I realize that the animals—chickens, pigs is what I recall— were available just to feed the household. There were no supermarkets, corner/neighborhood or convenience stores near the house. There was a store in town to buy food staples. I went there with cousins to get candy. This was when my grandparents were still living off the land not as farmers, but having a close connection to land for supplying most of their own food. I don't remember a garden though. That isn't to say that there wasn't one. It's just that at that time and even today, meat is the center of all meals. The other food—vegetables, potatoes, rice, etc. are considered side dishes—accompaniments.

Meat: The Center of Attention

In the American diet meat, considered a primary source of protein, is the main attraction around which side dishes revolve. I don't know when I first became aware of that fact, and the fact that food is essential to any social interaction. But there they are. Food can remain central to social situations, but as a society, we may want to rethink meat as a chief protein source in our diets and the focal point of all meals.

There is growing evidence that meat may play a significant role in the development of cancer and is likely a factor in premature aging. Early studies suggest that reduced animal protein intake may promote anti-cancer and anti-aging in humans.[32] Two new studies from different renowned, respected sources conclude meat consumption is linked to cancer risk. One study links the risk to how the meat is processed. The other study connects the risk to how the meat is

---

32   Long-term effects of calorie or protein restriction on serum 1GF-1 and 1GFBP-3 concentration in humans, Fontana L, et al, Division of Geriatrics and Nutritional Sciences, Washington University School of Medicine, St. Louis, MO 63110, LFontana@dom.wustl.edu.

cooked. In October 26, 2015 the World Health Organization released a report stating that red meats and processed meats are "carcinogenic to humans."[33] The University of Texas MD Anderson Cancer Center published a study released in early November 2015 that found diets high in meat may lead to increased risk of certain cancers created by cooking methods.[34]

Furthermore, according to Dr. Michael Greger, physician, author, and lecturer on public health issues, IGF-1 is released by our liver in response to animal protein consumption, regardless of how it's cooked.[35] Insulin-like Growth Factor – 1 or IGF-1 is a natural human growth hormone instrumental in normal growth during childhood, but in adulthood can promote abnormal growth—the proliferation, spread and invasion of cancer.[36]

We are bombarded with information on food and its connection to human health to the point of being overwhelmed, and confused. This information about IGF-1 and cancer from a couple of different sources got my attention. Like any theory, it warrants further study. However, it raises intriguing questions about how our body metabolizes animal protein, meat specifically. Until those questions are answered to my satisfaction, I chose to refrain from animal protein consumption.

Mystery Meat

Wild things

Apparently, my uncle knew someone who hunted. He himself didn't. To supplement food for our eight-person family, this acquaintance shared the rewards of a hunt with my uncle. Both freezers were full of hunted meat. For a number of Sunday dinners we were introduced to venison, rabbit and some other wild game. It was either buffalo or raccoon. As I remember the meat was seasoned and roasted. Although, how it was cooked didn't much matter. Serving the different meat types cut into

33   http://www.who.int/features/qa/cancer-red-meat/en/. Retrieved 10/26/2015.

34   http://www.mdanderson.org/newsroom/news-releases/2015/increased-meat-consumption-kidney-cancer-risk.html. Retrieved 11/8/2015.

35   Michael Greger, M.D., Estrogen in Cooked Meat, blog posted July 2, 2013.

36   www.nutritionfacts.org. Volume 10, September 25, 2012, Journal of Medicinal Food IGF-1 As One Stop Cancer Shops.

sections raised suspicion. The meat appeared dark, sinewy and generally unappetizing. It took me back to the flourless fried liver I prepared.

We generally ate our meals as a family at the kitchen table, all eight of us together. Special occasions and holidays were the exception. At those times, we gathered around the dining room table and used the "good china." I don't believe this was a holiday, but for sure being served such exotic fare was a special occasion. We were seated at the dining room table and used the good china. Looking back on it, the atmosphere of special occasion might have been a rouse to distract us from what was being served.

By this time, I might have been 15 or 16 years old. With nose wrinkled, furrowed brow, and referring to the meat in the center of the table, I asked the question, what is that? Without looking up from his meal my uncle replied tersely, it's chicken, eat it. But, of course, we knew it wasn't chicken. Presentation is half the battle in the serving of food. The meat looked horrible. I shudder to think about it. So we didn't eat it. We went to bed meatless that mystery meat night.

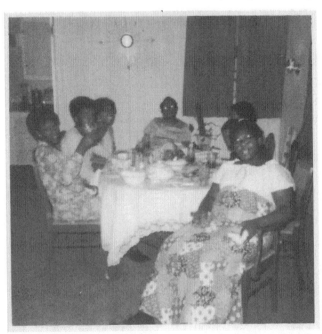

My sister Barbara in the glasses facing the camera. I'm on her left in the print dress glass raised, my boyfriend at the time seated to the left of me, cousin Joan, Aunt Ida, sister Diane and someone, probably either cousin Anita or Carl, behind Barbara – In the dining room Thanksgiving 1973.

Potted meat/Spam

As a member of the baby-boomers population, I was raised by the generation who lived through World War II and the Korean War. They were exposed to food scarcity. Potted meat was popularized during that time. My aunt and uncle kept a pantry full of canned food including potted meat, just in case. Potted meat is a term that describes different types of canned meat including Vienna sausages or miniature smoked sausage or weenies, and SPAM. Although SPAM has an identity of its own.

The term potted meat is strange—as if meat were planted in a pot, like flowers. Basically, it was. The type of meat was anyone's guess. It was likely meat from different parts of an animal probably pork, mashed together in salt and fat for a longer shelf life. It was pre-cooked so all you need do is open the can and eat from it. This went a long way in keeping people from going hungry during war time. Health wasn't a consideration.

Later as I understand it, potted meat was distributed as part of the U.S. government surplus food to poor families. This program pre-dated food stamps. We were recipients of this government food surplus. As children, particularly in our teen years, we never wanted to be associated with having received surplus food. Even though we ate it for breakfast with grits and eggs, for lunch as a sandwich, after-school for snack with saltine crackers, mixed with potatoes as hash, the meals derived from potted meat was endless.

Eating this way while we were young was harmless. Our bodies could process it. It is debatable whether the cumulative effect has an impact on middle-aged bodies. In other words, what we ate in our youth, haunts us in the form of deteriorating health as we get older. According to Dr. Weill, it may well have an impact. Eating that way at middle age and older is a heart attack waiting to happen. This next recipe is full of fiber and much more helpful to proper heart function.

Cabbage, Fennel and Kidney Beans

Preparation time: 15 minutes
Cooking time: 30 minutes
Serving size: 2

Ingredients:

2 Tbs. Olive oil
1 Cabbage, sliced
2 Fennel bulbs, sliced including tops
2 Tbs. Red pepper, crushed
1 Tbs. Black pepper, ground
2 Sweet potatoes, cubed
1 C. Red kidney beans, soaked and cooked
4 Green onions
1 C. Vegetable stock

Directions:

In a medium sauté skillet, heat olive oil, then add fennel and cook until caramelized. Add onions, stir and cook until translucent. The caramelized fennel will give the dish a sweet note in addition to its unique licorice taste to complement the savory beans and potatoes. Stir in cabbage, add seasoning and cook until cabbage is wilted. Add beans and vegetable broth. Cook until broth has nearly disappeared. Let stand for 5 minutes before serving.

The Headless Chicken

"Running around like a chicken with its head cut off" was more than just an expression one day at our house on St. Clair and Tremont Streets. I don't know if it was inspiration from our visit with Grandma and having a fresh chicken for dinner or what, but Mother brought home a live chicken from a Public Market shopping trip.

The Public Market is Rochester's version of a farmers' market. I don't remember how she got that live bird home. She didn't own a car and relied on public transportation, or the goodness of friends and neighbors to get around. Anyway, she somehow managed to get the live bird home. The next thing I knew, Mother cut off its head.

But before she could put it into a pan and cover it like grandpa did, the headless bird went running wildly around the kitchen, blood spurting and splattering everywhere. The bird followed my screaming sister and me out the side door from the kitchen. It was Mr. Bannister who came to the rescue.

Mr. Bannister was the neighbor across the street whose house was kitty-corner to ours. I don't know if he heard our screams or if mother sought him out but he knew to come help catch the headless bird. He caught the chicken, wrung what remained of its neck and brought it back to mother's kitchen. The rest of that evening is a blank in my memory. As traumatic as that experience was, it somehow didn't turn me against eating meat. In fact, I liked chicken. I ate it after that incident and up until 2013. But as poultry goes, I loved, loved, loved turkey, and still do. I just can't eat it anymore.

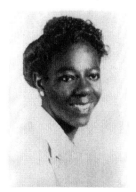

My mother, Tryphena as a young woman,
way before the headless chicken incident.

Meat doesn't have to dominate meals. The recipes that follow place plant-based food at the center of the meal. I find them hearty enough that those of you accustomed to meat won't miss it.

Spinach, Mushroom, Garlic Marinara Sauce over White Quinoa

Preparation time: 10 minutes
Cooking time: 25 minutes
Serving size: 2

Ingredients:

2 Tbs. Olive oil
⅓ C. Crimini mushrooms, sliced
3 Tbs. Red pepper, crushed
½ lbs Spinach
½ lbs Basil
1 Yellow onion, sliced

1–16 oz. Marinara sauce, garlic flavored
½ C. White wine
2 C. Vegetable broth
1 C. White Quinoa

Directions:

In a medium sauce pan, cook quinoa according to package directions. Instead of water, use vegetable broth. Set the cooked quinoa aside to cool.

While the quinoa is cooking, heat olive oil in a medium size non-stick skillet. Slice onion. Place mushrooms in the heated oil. Let them simmer over low to medium flame until they cook down creating mushroom juice. Add sliced onions and cook until translucent. When the onions are cooked, add marinara sauce, wine and crushed red pepper. Let the mixture simmer for 10 - 15 minutes. Stir occasionally. Add spinach and basil to the mixture simmering only until the leaves are slightly wilted yet bright green.

Serve:

Spoon quinoa onto a plate; ladle the sauce over the quinoa and let the dish rest for 1 minute before serving.

The Great Outdoors

Picnics

Picnics were a big production in our household. They always took place in a public park. Picnicking in a park distinguished it from a barbecue, which took place in the backyard of the house on Grand Avenue. Picnics happened mostly during summer holidays. Occasionally, they would be a summer surprise. My uncle was usually the organizer. He developed the menu. It was always the same—barbecue pork ribs, hamburgers, hot dogs, potato salad, baked beans, Cole slaw, corn-on-the-cob, a watermelon or two, chips and dip. The dip was always French onion. He would invite loads of friends and family. Sometimes he'd ask them to bring dishes from the menu. Whether they did or not, my uncle would always have that dish on hand.

Preparing for the picnic began the night before. My aunt made the barbecue sauce from scratch. Making the sauce the night before gives the ingredients time for the flavors to blend for a full flavor. I find that to be true with most recipes. It's why leftovers taste so good the next day. Potato salad is a make-ahead dish that can be refrigerated overnight. Also the night before, pork ribs were parboiled or baked to reduce the fat. Parboiling also reduced time and flare-ups on the grill.

On picnic day, someone from the family would rise early to stake out our place in the park. We had to have several grills—one to cook the ribs, the other to cook the hamburgers and hot dogs we'd have for lunch while the ribs were cooking, a shelter with plenty of picnic tables for the food, but also the pinochle or bid whist card games that would go on most of the day. There had to be a place for the kids to play kick ball or some other ball game and a playground area. We were a bit demanding. To make sure we had everything we needed to both enjoy the outdoors and have the comforts of home, we packed and loaded into the car all we could think of for a day in the park. There were pots, roasting pans, bowls, metal cooking utensils including spatulas, spoons, tongs, forks, knives, (we gave a whole new meaning to the expression everything but the kitchen sink) charcoal, lighter fluid, paper plates, plastic cups, eating utensils, table cloths, blankets, dish towels and rags, ice—there was never enough ice, someone was always sent on an ice run, cards, balls, water guns, balloons (a water balloon war was always a possibility). This is what it took for us to eat alfresco in a public park. Talk about a production! Inevitably, we'd end up bringing the ribs home because by dark they were either still under cooked (even with the pre-cooking) or they were overcooked to the point of charring and no one wanted them. Below are a few recipes that pay homage to our family picnics but are plant-based and of lighter fare.

Cole Slaw

Preparation time: 30 minutes
Cooking time: 20 minutes
Serving size: 12

Ingredients:

Cole Slaw
½ Green Cabbage, medium-size,
    shredded
½ Red Cabbage, shredded
4 Carrots, shredded
2 Yellow/brown Onion, sliced
1½ C. Golden Raisins
1 C. Pineapple Chunks

Dressing
¼ C. Honey
½ C. Apple Cider Vinegar
4 Tsp. Ginger, minced [optional]
½ C. Pineapple Juice

Directions:

Cole Slaw Direction: Combine slaw ingredients in a large mixing bowl. Thoroughly mix ingredients to evenly distribute for flavor and appearance.

*Dressing Directions:*Mix honey and vinegar together. Add ginger if you prefer. To the honey, vinegar mixture add pineapple juice until syrupy.

Drizzle the dressing over the slaw ingredients. Mix the ingredients together until they are well coated. Refrigerate for about 1 hour.

Serve:

This makes a great side dish at any picnic.

Girl Scout Camp

We were involved in Girl Scouts from Brownies through to Cadets. We went to scout meetings Wednesday's after school. We walked from our house to the Mount Olivet Baptist Church basement for the meetings. No one walks any more. Nowadays, parents usually drive the kids to their extracurricular activities and there's a schedule. Back then, in the early 60s, kids walked. We walked great distances. Walked from our apartment to pick up our cousins at least three miles away. From there we wound our way to the church another four or five miles. It was me, my sister Diane, and two cousins.

Our troop leaders were Miss Dorothy Kensington for Brownies, and Mrs. Lydia Clayton for Cadets. They were Mount Olivet Church members which is why we were able to meet in the church basement. Miss Kensington was in her 40s or 50s, but looked older. She was average height, about 5' 4" or 5' 5". She had a dark complexion, and wore her short, thinning hair straightened. She had a round figure with a protruding tummy. The Brownie leader uniform didn't do a thing for her. Miss Kensington wore glasses, with thick prescription lenses. I don't think she was married. I know she was childless. The scouts became her children. I remember hearing that she was a nurse by profession. She had a gentle way about her, but don't get her angry. She could be very stern and didn't tolerate foolishness.

I didn't like the Brownie uniform. It was a 1-piece, belted brown dress and came with a little brown beanie cap. Didn't do a thing for me either. I was glad to advance to the Cadet level where the uniform was more stylish. The Cadet uniform was a green two-piece with a sash worn across the shoulder for your pins and a cute green barrette.

I liked the name Lydia, my Cadet leader's name. Thought I'd name my daughter Lydia. But I never had a daughter. Mrs. Clayton was tall— maybe 5' 7" or 5' 8". At least that's the way she seemed to a 12-year old. She was light-skinned and wore her hair just below her ears, short and straight. Straight was the fashion. Afro's hadn't caught on yet with the older generation. She might have been about the same age as Miss Kensington. Mrs. Clayton was married and had two daughters. They were older and not part of our Cadet troop. Mrs. Clayton also had a gentle demeanor. She spoke softly and was very patient. I don't know what her profession was or if she had a profession or worked at all. I don't ever remember seeing her angry.

I used to love to go to Girl Scouts. It was a way to get out of the house for few hours and maybe learn something new and different. We learned how to make placemats and seat cushions out of newspapers. I can still make them. You never know when you might need to make placemats or seat cushions. We also made lanyards for holding keys. Someday when the world has collapsed into itself due to either a natural or man-made disaster of some kind, having those skills I learned in Girl Scouts will come in handy. Anyway, what I liked most about Girl Scouts was overnight camping in the woods. We were able to get away for a few days not just a few hours. It was glorious.

There was the bus ride to the camp site in the Adirondack Mountains. We learned camp songs along the way. We slept in raised tents with netting to keep out the bugs and critters. I loved the smell of the pine and sage of the woods. We brought sleeping bags. If we didn't have commercial sleeping bags, and we didn't, we learned how to make them from blankets.

We laid out the blankets fully, layered them one on the other. We then folded them in half length-wise, one inside the other. Once the blankets were folded, we placed our clothes and other belongings like flashlights, bug spray etc. on the folded blankets. Then we rolled them up from the bottom and folded the ends inside for easy carrying.

Once at the camp grounds, we were assigned our tents. They were equipped with bunk beds, each with a mattress. Our sleeping "bags" were the linen. There were different activities most to teach us how to be independent, self-sufficient in the rawest most basic circumstances. We were assigned or volunteered to do different tasks—cooking, dish washing, wood gathering for campfires, camp grounds clean up including the latrines. We usually took turns doing different chores. We sang Taps at the end of the day:

Day is done,
Gone the sun
From the lake, from the hills, from the sky,
All is well, safely rest
God is nigh.

At least I think that is the last line of the song. Taps, as you know, is part of solemn military funerals. Always performed by a lone bugler. You never hear the lyrics. I was proud to know (for the most part) and be able to sing the lyrics to Taps. Reveille was the song to start the day, but thank goodness for you, I don't know the words.

Cooking was one of the chores I liked doing. I remember pancake breakfasts. Preparing the pots by rubbing liquid dish detergent on the bottom to guard against them burning on the open flame. For lunch or dinner, there was baked beans, corn on the cob, probably hot dogs. Cooking the hot dogs over an open fire was fun. We'd find long sticks, sharpen the ends on a rock, and stick the hot dog on the sharpened end to place over the flame until it was toasty or charred, whichever came first. We toasted marshmallows the same way.

Then there were the S'mores. You know, the marshmallow, milk chocolate (Hershey's) melted between two graham crackers. It was a great camp out dessert. Although I pledge this book is focused on main dishes, it's hard not to include this favorite campfire dessert when discussing camping. Overnight camping was my first experience with S'mores.

S'mores

Preparation time: 10 minutes
Cooking time: 5-7 minutes
Serving size: 12

Ingredients:

1 – Package of marshmallows
12 Milk chocolate bars (Hershey)
1 box Graham crackers

Directions:

If you're in the great outdoors camping, collect medium round, long tree twigs. With a pocket knife, whittle away one end of the twig to make a sharp point. Or you can use a smooth stone or rock to rub the end of the twig to make a sharp point, rotating each side until it is sharpened. If you're in your backyard, use long skewer sticks soaked in water. Pierce the marshmallow with the stick point. With the other end of the stick, hold the marshmallow over an open fire until it becomes golden on most sides. Have the mild chocolate bars on half of a graham cracker ready to place the melted, hot marshmallow on top. Cover the marshmallow with the other half of a graham cracker to make a kind of sandwich and let it sit for the chocolate to soften and the marshmallow cools enough to bite into this gooey treat. A guilty pleasure over the top sugar. This makes a great end of the day dessert every blue moon.

Baked Beans

Preparation time: 5 minutes
Cooking time: 2 hours
Serving size: 8

Ingredients:

2 C. Small White Beans (soaked)
2 Tbs. Liquid smoke
1½ C. Molasses
4 C. Water

Directions:

In a medium sauce pan, place the beans in water and cook on the stove over high heat until the water boils. Turn the heat to simmer and cook the beans for 45 minutes. Add molasses and liquid smoke. Bring the beans to a boil again, reduce the flame to simmer and cook for another 45 minutes or until beans are tender. Stir occasionally to prevent beans from sticking to the bottom of the pan. As the beans cook, they will take on the color of the molasses and soften in syrup composed of both molasses and juice derived from the cooked beans. Place the bean mixture in a baking dish and bake at 325 degrees for 1/2 hour until bubbly. Remove the dish from the oven and let stand for 5 minutes before serving.

Barbecues

Barbecues in the backyard at Grand Avenue weren't as big a production as picnics, but a production nonetheless. Inherent in the barbecue is grilling of meat over an open fire. Usually it was pork or beef ribs, sometimes chicken, hamburgers and hot dogs. My uncle's grill was made from an old oil barrel, cut lengthwise in half and hinged together. The bottom half was fitted with a wire rack where the food was placed with space under the rack for charcoal. The top half was used as a cover for smoking the food (meat). A handle was placed on the outside of the top portion for convenience in raising and lowering the cover.

Water balloon wars were no stranger to our backyard barbecues. The "yard" was mainly asphalt. The driveway emptied into the backyard. On barbecue days, no one was allowed to park in the backyard. The asphalt took up about 85% of the backyard. Curving to the right of the asphalt was a grassy area. It covered about 8 feet with rose bushes marking the property line to the far right. At the end of the asphalt was a 4-car garage. Two of the garages housed cars. The other two were for storage. Tools, gardening supplies and miscellaneous stuff could be found there. From the back porch one could see this site. There were no trees blocking the view or for hiding from water balloon enemies.

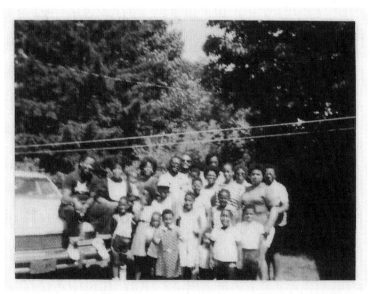

The bunch of us at a family barbecue in the backyard on Grand Avenue, July 1982. I'm on the left in red near back row.

Grilled Summer Vegetables

Preparation time: 15 minutes
Cooking time: 10 minutes
Serving size: 6-8

Ingredients:

Corn kernels (organic) – if the cob is preferred, these can be grilled separately
Portobello mushroom, (large, whole)
Yellow squash, cut into medallions
Red bell pepper, quartered
Carrots, cut into medallions
Eggplant, sliced width-wise
Yellow Onion, sliced
Olive oil
Balsamic vinaigrette

Directions:

Use a sharp knife to shave corn kernels from the cob into a large bowl. Cut the squash, carrots, eggplant and onion into medallions about 1/2 inch thick. Place them into the bowl with the corn. The bell pepper can be quartered and joined with the other vegetables. Add the olive oil and balsamic vinaigrette to the cut vegetables and mix well. They are now ready for grilling.

The mushrooms should remain whole. They can be brushed with olive oil and vinaigrette. Mushrooms may be placed directly on the grill grate. They may take extra time to grill until tender.

Meanwhile, the cut vegetables can be grilled together placed into a special vegetable holder for grilling or wrapped in aluminum foil and placed on the grill. Either way, they will take about 10 minutes to become tender and flavorful depending on the thickness of their cut.

Serve:

Immediately after removing them from the grill. Cooking the vegetables in this way somehow unleashes a brighter flavor from each of the vegetables giving the diner a different taste experience from the familiar.

Skewer Grilled Vegetables and Garlic Marinade

Preparation time: 30 minutes
Cooking time: 10-15 minutes
Serving size: 8-10

Ingredients:

4 Yellow squash, medium-size	*Marinade*
2 Fennel bulbs	1 Lemon
4 Red bell pepper	4 Garlic cloves
2 Yellow onion, large	2 Tbs. Honey
1 Eggplant, medium size	1 Tbs. Olive Oil
1 pint Crimini mushrooms, whole	2 Tbs. Chives
4 Carrots	¼ Tsp. Black pepper, coarse

Directions:

Soak 10-12 bamboo skewers in water for about an hour in preparation for grilling. This will prevent the skewers from burning.

Wash all the vegetables thoroughly. Dry the mushrooms. Cut the squash and carrots into 1/2 inch medallions. Remove the green stalks from the fennel and the bottom of the fennel bulb. Cut the fennel bulbs into quarters and separate each piece from the bulb. Quarter the bell pepper. Width-wise cut the pepper in half. Remove remaining seeds and inner membrane. Quarter the onion. With the skin on, cut the eggplant into chunks. Cut the mushrooms in half. Set the vegetables aside until the skewers are soaked.

To make the marinade, juice the lemon into a medium mixing bowl. Mince the garlic and add it to the lemon juice. Add honey, olive oil and black pepper. Finely chop the chives and add them to the mixture along with a zest of the lemon. Whisk the ingredients until they are well blended and set the marinade aside while the skewers are assembled.

To assemble the skewers, beginning with the eggplant, add red bell pepper, fennel, squash, carrot, onion, mushroom, and end with the eggplant. Assemble all the skewers until all the vegetables are used. Place them in a shallow dish.

Drizzle the marinade over the vegetables and refrigerate for about 30 minutes until ready for grilling. Grill until the vegetables are tender and serve.

Serve:

Any remaining marinade can be drizzled over vegetables on the serving dish.

Snuffy's aka Smittey's

I don't know how Snuffy got his nickname. That's how he was known in the Black community. But his name was Smith. Thus Smittey's the name on his restaurant. His place had cornbread and beans as side orders. However, Snuffy's was celebrated for its chicken wings and ribs.

What distinguished Snuffy's wings and ribs from all others was the sauce. He called the sauce he invented his Boss Sauce. It was absolutely boss. There is nothing else like it in the world. The sauce combines sweetness, hot chili heat, and tang. At least at Snuffy's a vegetable was part of the menu. He offered creamy cole slaw made with shredded cabbage, carrots and either pineapple or golden raisins and lots of mayonnaise.

Snuffy's place was mostly for take-out orders. There were just a few tables for dining in. Friday and Saturday nights you couldn't get near the place. There were lines of people snaking out the door and down the street waiting to place an order. It didn't matter what you ordered, as long as it was drenched in boss sauce. Bet it would be great on grilled vegetables like Portobello mushrooms. The following barbecue sauce recipe isn't Boss Sauce, but it's good on grilled vegetables and fish.

Barbecue Sauce

Preparation time: 20 minutes
Cooking time: 90 minutes
Serving size: 8

Ingredients:

4 C. Tomato sauce
½ C. Mustard, spiced or brown
1 C. Bourbon
1 Tbs. Horseradish
4 Tbs. Garlic, minced
¼ C. Molasses

¼ C. Apple Cider Vinegar
½ C. Worcestershire Sauce
1 Tsp. Cayenne pepper
1 Tsp. Black pepper
1 Tbs. Olive Oil, extra virgin

Directions:

In a Dutch oven or stock pot, mix the ingredients together. Simmer the mixed ingredients over medium to low flame for about 90 minutes or until the sauce thickens. I find this to be the right combination of sweet, savory and spicing ingredients to complement especially Portobello mushrooms, haddock and cod fish. When it reaches the desired thickness remove the sauce from the heat. It is ready to coat over your choice of vegetables or fish.

Clambakes

Growing up in the northeast where there are four seasons, the fall season was generally reserved for clambakes. Our uncle really intended for us to be exposed to as much new and different kinds of experiences and foods as possible. Seafood was part of that different experience. As the weather cooled down, our food menu turned from light dishes like salads and quick prepared foods to heavier, hearty dishes that took time to cook like stews and soups. One of my favorite stew-like dishes was the food we had at clambakes.

We were first exposed to clambakes through our church—Trinity Presbyterian. Every fall, usually in October, our church would hold a clambake as its annual fundraiser. The clambakes were held in a cabin at a park. My uncle was on the clambake committee. The menu consisted of chicken, sweet potatoes, white potatoes, corn-on-the-cob, cole slaw and dozens and dozens of clams. All ingredients except for the cole slaw were scrubbed clean and boiled together in one big pot. Potatoes were cooked with their skins on. Occasionally, lobster or shrimp were added. The mingling of flavors from each ingredient created a wonderful broth. I believe the broth may have had medicinal benefits. Or maybe it just made you feel good and warm inside on a crisp autumn day in the park. Each family bought clambake dinners and sold tickets to other family and friends to benefit the church. It was at one of the clambakes that I decided I had a crush on one of the boys—Nathaniel.

Nathaniel and I were the same age. He was in my Sunday school class. Our teacher was Mrs. Coles. Mrs. Coles had a daughter, Natalie who wasn't in our class but I mention because her name would become famous. No, she's not that Natalie Cole.

I liked Nathaniel because he was shy, and had a low-key personality. He was light-skinned, had a long face and a nice smile with teeth that protruded a bit as if he sucked his thumb. He was always friendly towards me which was unusual at the time for light-skinned boys to be friendly and interested in dark-skinned girls and vice versa. There was this unspoken but prominent divide between light-skinned and dark-skinned Blacks. Our attraction in spite of the common practice could be because we were just 10 or 11 years old and were as yet unaffected by this strange intra-racial splintering. Nathaniel went to a different public school than I, so we only saw each other on Sundays. That could be why I liked him, because in my own shyness he was a safe distance from me and we didn't have to interact often.

While the food was cooking, there would be games like horse shoes, badminton, or cards to play. In my mind, Nathaniel and I would skip the games to go for long walks in the park and talk instead. The fallen leaves with all their beautiful bright colors would crunch under our feet as we walked. Our conversations were about nothing in particular, but they were private and we didn't want our younger sisters following us, listening in. Which they always tried to do. In reality, although I don't know how it happened but at some point, he took my telephone number. When he called and he was announced because someone other than me answered the phone, my family began to tease me.

When the church clambakes ended, my uncle would organize a clambake for family and friends. Always in the fall, always held in a cabin, in a park. It was like a potluck, with each family bringing a dish or ingredient from the agreed upon menu. In a good financial year, shrimp and/or a lobster or two would be added. The following recipes remind me of those days.

Steamed Clams

Preparation time: 10 minutes
Cooking time: 15 minutes
Serving size: 4

Ingredients:

¼ C. Non-dairy butter
4 Tbs. Garlic, minced
¼ C. Apple cider vinegar
4 C. Water
2 Tbs. Coriander
2 Tbs. Cumin

¼ C. Parsley, finely chopped
½ C. Celery, chopped
2 Doz. Clams, medium cherry-stone
1 Crusted bread loaf

Directions:

In a heated Dutch oven melt butter and add garlic. Once the garlic and butter is heated over low heat add water, cider vinegar, parsley, coriander, and cumin. When the mixture bubbles, add clams and celery and stir. Cover the pan and steam the clams until they open. Be sure to ladle the seasoned liquid over the open clams.

Cut the bread loaf length-wise in half. Spread butter generously over the loaf. Once the butter is spread, spread minced garlic over the butter. If you have garlic butter use it instead. Toast the bread until it is golden brown.

Serve:

In a deep dish place the clams, ladle the liquid over them. Squeeze lemon over the open clams. Serve with a hearty piece of toasted crusted garlic bread.

Cabbage & Shrimp

Preparation time: 10 minutes
Cooking time: 45 minutes
Serving size: 4

Ingredients:

1 Cabbage head, green, shredded
1 Onion, yellow, sliced
2 Tbs. Red pepper, crushed
2 Tbs. Black pepper, ground
½ lbs Shrimp, medium size, cooked

1 Sweet potato, peeled and cubed
¼ C. Vegetable broth
2 Tbs. Olive oil

Directions:

In a medium sauce pan, heat olive oil. Add onion and sauté until caramelized. Add shredded cabbage to the onion and simmer until cabbage is wilted. Gradually stir in vegetable broth as juices from the cabbage evaporate. Add crushed red pepper and black pepper. Stir to mix onion, cabbage and seasonings. Add sweet potato and cook until the largest potato chunk can be pierced with a fork. Stir in shrimp during the last 5 minutes of cooking.

These next two recipes are among my favorites. I cook them frequently. They are great tasting meals that can be made lightning fast during a work week.

Snow Peas, Mushrooms & Garbanzo Beans

Preparation time: 5 minutes (not including the beans)
Cooking time: 15 minutes
Serving size: 2

Ingredients:

1 lbs Snow peas
1/3 C Crimini mushrooms, sliced
1 C. Garbanzo beans, soaked, cooked

1 Tbs. Garlic, minced
2 Tbs. Olive oil
¼ C. Vegetable broth, organic, low-sodium

Directions:

Soak beans for a minimum of 3 hours before cooking. This can be done the night before to have them ready for cooking.

Cover soaked garbanzo beans with vegetable broth in a saucepan, add garlic and cook the beans until nearly tender. Set them aside.

In a medium sauté pan heat the olive oil. Add mushrooms, cover the pan and simmer until golden brown. The mushrooms

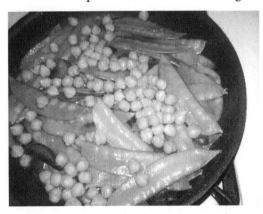

make their own earthy flavored juice or pot liquor. Stir in snow peas and cook until tender. Add cooked garbanzo beans and remaining garlic seasoned vegetable broth. Simmer until liquid just covers the bottom of the pan. They are ready to serve.

Pan Sautéed Salmon with Spinach

Preparation time: 5 minutes
Cooking time: 15 minutes
Serving size: 2

Ingredients:

2 Wild Salmon Filets
2 lb. Fresh Spinach
2 Tbs. Olive Oil
¼ C. Garlic Butter
1 Lemon

4 Garlic Cloves, minced
¼ Tsp. Nutmeg
¼ Tsp. Turmeric
¼ Tsp. Black Pepper, coarsely
ground

With the controversy now surrounding salmon, it's best to buy wild salmon rather than farm raised salmon. With farm raised salmon you risk them being GMO.

Directions:

In a 10" sauté pan, heat 2 tablespoon of olive oil. Wash the salmon filets and pat dry with a clean towel. Squeeze 1/4 lemon over each side of the salmon for both filets. Spread softened garlic butter over both sides of each of the salmon filets. Sprinkle pepper on the filets to cover both sides. Place the salmon into the heated pan skin side down and cook uncovered until browned about 3 minutes. Flip the salmon and cook until flaky.

Remove the salmon and set aside to rest. In the same sauté pan add another tablespoon of olive oil and remaining garlic butter. Add spinach and stir in the minced garlic. Sprinkle in nutmeg and turmeric while stirring the spinach. Cook until the spinach is tender about 5 minutes. Just before removing the spinach from the flame, squeeze a lemon quarter over the spinach. The added lemon brightens the flavor combinations.

Serve:

Plate the dish with spinach serving as a bed to the salmon fillets.

Passages

When my mother died, I remember the house filling up with people. They brought casseroles and baking dishes of food. There were tuna casseroles, made with different kinds of pasta, and Italian-style lasagna in the casserole category. It seems no matter what the racial, cultural background, when there's a death, friends always bring food to the family. It's a practice that ensures the family has nourishment while not having to concern themselves with meal preparation. The family has the space to grieve and to deal with the practical matters of funeral arrangements and caring for those left behind. Bringing food gives friends the feeling of having provided practical support instead of feeling helplessness at an emotionally stressful time.

Upon learning of my mother's death and the realization of what that meant, I went numb. Traumatized by this sudden, enormous loss took away all my feelings, hunger included. I wouldn't allow myself to feel anything. I went through the motions of having food in front of me and pretending to eat, but it would be days before my appetite returned. When it did, it was the classic comfort food macaroni & cheese that I craved. The following recipe is a quick, easy, and hearty plant-based alternative to the dairy and carbohydrate-laden casseroles as a dish to support a grieving family.

This full-flavored dish contains antioxidants in broccoli and tomatoes as well as the anti-inflammatory turmeric spice. Broccoli is one of those vegetables with a strong, bitter taste. I've tried different ingredients to tone down the bitterness including nutmeg but nothing seemed to work except tomatoes. On a tip given to me, I add tomatoes to meals with broccoli and voilà, the bitterness is less pronounced. Unless you like the bitterness, try adding tomatoes and see what you think. Tomatoes also give the dish a more colorful appearance. Fiber of the broccoli and beans enriches this dish with heartiness that holds off hunger for hours.

Broccoli, Mushrooms & Stewed Tomatoes

Preparation time: 10 minutes
Cooking time: 20 minutes
Serving size: 4

Ingredients:

1 C Crimini Mushrooms, sliced
2 Tbs. Garlic, minced
16 oz. Broccoli florets
8 oz. Stewed tomatoes

¼ C Great Northern Navy beans,
   soaked, cooked
2 Tbs. Olive oil
½ Tbs. Turmeric

Directions:

In a sauté pan heat olive oil, then add mushrooms. Cover the pan and cook until mushrooms are browned and release their liquid. Blend in minced garlic until heated through. Add broccoli to the pan and cook for about 1 minute. Fold in stewed tomatoes, and turmeric. Simmer until the florets are tender. Mix in the Navy beans with the pot liquor they generated for more flavor in the last 5 minutes of cooking.

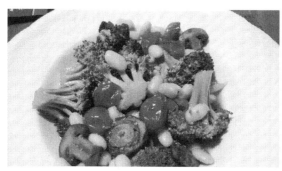

Our Relationship with Food

Our relationship with food has changed over time. We still understand how essential it is to our existence, but we don't treat it with the reverence it deserves as some cultures still do. Eat to exist, as Dr. Joel Fuhrman urges us to do in his book Eat to Live (Fuhrman 2003, 2011) has become "exist to eat." With that approach, one would think food is the focus of our lives, instead it has become an accompaniment. While food is key to our social interactions, we take food for granted. It is almost part of the background noise, if you will. Comfort food has entered into our consciousness and lexicon recently. Depending on whom you ask, comfort food can be described as that food that makes us feel good, reminds us of good times. It is an emotional association with food. Heavy, substantial dishes like macaroni and cheese, almost any pasta dish in fact, as well as dishes involving stews, and roasts might all be considered comfort food. It is food we use to fill an emotional void. Food consumed for this reason should raise red flags.

Foods we have eaten over time in some ways reflects the maturity of our palates. As young children the simpler the food the better. Bean 'n' franks, spaghetti and meatballs were enough. As we age and our palates become more sophisticated we were ready for more complex foods and dining. When people are asked why they eat or what food does for them, they most likely respond, I eat because I'm hungry or food satisfies my hunger. The answer is rarely associated with food providing nourishment or energy. Hunger is a signal to your brain that the body has run out of fuel or energy to keep it going. Instead of looking for fresh, nourishing food to keep us going, we settle for processed food with no nutrient value that tastes good but makes us lethargic and only generates small spurts of energy. We can have great tasting, richly nutritious food that ingested moderately gives us long-lasting energy. That's what this book is about.

Super-size is another relatively new term associated with food. First introduced in the fast food retail arena in the 1980s and 1990s, it quickly spilled over into the sit-down restaurant world with the competitiveness of the food retail industry and low profit margins. Super-size could be described as single portion sizes large enough to feed a family of four. Typically, those portions are consumed by a single person compelled to finish it in one meal whether they felt full with a quarter of the portion consumed or not.

The clean plate club was a concept perpetuated by our uncle and aunt and probably most parents and guardians who grew up during war when food was scarce. The idea was to protect us from their war-like experience, and starvation or the threat of it. Joining the clean plate club meant eating every morsel on your plate whether you were full or not, until the plate was completely empty or clean. After all, there were children in Africa starving was the familiar refrain. You were made to feel guilty about not eating everything put before you. For many of us, that orientation never left us as adults. We are compelled to eat all that we are served. Combine the clean plate club with this super-sized food environment means consumption of more food in one meal than we really need. We have to re-orient ourselves for improved health and better quality of life as we age.

Native American and Asian cultures, particularly the Japanese, view food with respect as a means of sustenance. For those cultures, there's a recognition that some living thing, plant or animal, is sacrificed so that we humans might live. They only take what is needed to live and no more. Many of these cultures have rituals to honor the life taken for our nourishment. Where animals are concerned, we lessen the harsh reality of animal slaughter by placing middlemen between the killing of an animal and the cooking and eating of its carcass. We buy meat nicely packaged in the supermarket ready for cooking and don't have to concern ourselves with how it got there. I promised not to go too deeply into the morals and ethics of meatless eating, but will leave this thought— if we took time to consider where our food comes from, and those responsible for getting it to us, we might treat it with more respect, be grateful for our food source, and more thoughtful about what we put into our bodies and why. No one is immune to the harmful effects of an unhealthy relationship with food and its consequences on human health. Celebrities with more financial resources than the average person have also suffered diet-related casualties. We lost many talented people prematurely including the following that stood out for me—-Grammy award winning vocal artist and songwriter, Luther Vandross, died at age 54 of complications from a stroke. He was diabetic. We all watched as his weight yo-yo'd up and down within short spans of time before his stroke. Fannie Lou Hamer, civil rights activist who coined the phrase *I'm sick and tired of being sick and tired* as she fought for voting rights in the segregated south and equal representation among the Mississippi delegation to the 1960 Democratic National Convention, succumbed to heart failure at age 59. Cass Elliott of the 1960s Mommas & the Pappas, died at the age of 32 of a heart attack. She was obese. Karen Carpenter of the singing duo the Carpenters died at age 32 of heart failure after combatting anorexia nervosa for eight years. Rap artist Heavy D died from pulmonary embolism. He had heart disease, which was also believed to be a contributing factor in his death. He was 44 years old and obese. An unhealthy relationship with food is no joke.

In some ways food becomes an extension of our identity. Food represents our racial or geographic origins—Italian, French, Swedish, Irish, Soul Food is usually associated with Southern African-American dishes, New Orleans—Creole and Cajun, etc. Family identity is sometimes tied up with recipes handed down for generations—pies, breads, pastries of all sorts like tarts, turnovers for example. Personal identity with certain specific dishes associated with the family member who perfected it...Mama's tamales, Grandma's potato salad, Aunt Ruth's sweet potato pie, etc. In these examples, recipes become sacred. Only a select few know the original recipe and are sworn to secrecy. Although the recipe may use ingredients that are now considered unhealthful, no one dares update it for fear of being accused of committing a sacrilegious act or at the very least insulting the ethnic origins from which the recipe was derived or family tradition. If lives are to be spared preventable food-related disease and premature death, that mindset must be re-examined.

We baby boomers are the generation that shook-up traditions in the late 1950s and 1960s. We questioned the status quo. That questioning gave birth to the civil rights movement, the woman's movement, gay rights and all their attending issues. Even as we age, we continue to question what is acceptable and create the new normal in all aspects of our life including food, especially as we learn the effects food has on our bodies. We grow more mature in our knowledge of the food/body connection, we free ourselves from the outdated beliefs and practices that give rise to premature aging and death.

Stuffed Bell Peppers

Preparation time: 30 minutes
Cooking time: 45 minutes
Serving size: 4

Ingredients:

½ C. Tri-color Quinoa
½ Yellow onion, medium-size, diced
4 Tbs. Garlic, minced
2 Celery stalks, sliced bite-size
½ C. Sesame Seeds, toasted (optional – any nut can be used like walnuts, pecans, almonds)

4 Bell peppers (red, yellow, green)
1½ C. Vegetable broth, organic
4 Tbs. Garlic Powder
2 Tbs. Black pepper, ground
4 Tbs. Olive oil

Directions:

In a quart sized sauce pan, pour 1 cup vegetable broth. Place the pan on a high flame. Bring the broth to a boil. Add 1/2 cup tri-colored quinoa and garlic, stir until the quinoa is covered and the garlic disappears. Bring the mixture to a boil in the uncovered sauce pan. Reduce the flame to low. Cover the pan and let the mixture simmer until the moisture completely absorbed. Remove the pan from the flame and let the quinoa stand.

While the quinoa is cooking, toast the seeds or nuts in 1 tablespoon of olive oil. Remove the toasted nuts into a separate dish to cool. Dice and slice the onion and celery. Sauté the onion and celery in 1 tablespoon of olive oil until translucent. Remove from the flame and let the vegetables rest. In a large mixing bowl, place the quinoa, toasted seeds or nuts, onion and celery. Add the black pepper and garlic powder. Stir the mixture together adding 1/4 cup of vegetable broth.

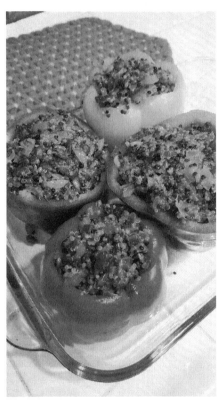

Let the mixture stand while preparing the bell peppers. Remove the top of the bell pepper by cutting a circle around the stem. Remove the top and from the top remove the seeds inside until the cavity is completely empty, rinse. Rub any remaining olive oil on the outside of the bell peppers. Into the empty bell pepper cavity, scoop the quinoa mixture into the peppers until all are filled.

Place the filled peppers upright into a shallow baking dish. Add any remaining vegetable broth to the baking dish. Cover the baking dish and bake for 30 minutes. Remove the covering and bake for another 10-15 minutes until the peppers are tender and the filling is browned.

Serve:

Let the stuffed peppers rest for 5 minutes before serving.

The filling for peppers can be prepared up to 1 day before serving. Seasoned cooks know preparing ahead of serving not only cuts down on your time in the kitchen, but also gives the ingredients a chance to mingle for richer flavor.

Dining Out

My first experience at fine dining was as a 17-year old high school junior. My first boyfriend exposed me to Mandarin Chinese cuisine. Our date was dinner at Cathay Pagoda on Main Street in Rochester, New York. The exterior of the restaurant had a pagoda façade. I remember yellow and red trim. When you enter the restaurant you see the maître d station in the foyer. Bamboo curtains separate the foyer from the dining area. There are two or three sections of seating area. The restaurant is dimly lit with Chinese lanterns and colorful parasols turned upside down make up the ceiling. The maître d, who was also the owner, greeted us warmly and seated us at a table for two tucked away in a corner. I felt special. We were always well dressed. Rather sophisticated young adults. My boyfriend had a lot to do with me feeling special, but the restaurant owner played a role too.

The owner was a flamboyant Chinese woman usually dressed in a satin, form-fitting mandarin-style dress that buttoned on the side ending at the top of her mandarin-collar with splits on the side exposing her model/dancer legs to mid-thigh. She was heavily made up. Black eyeliner flared out past the corners of her eyes and up towards her thin, arched eyebrows. She wore green or blue eye shadow, bright red lips and rosy high cheek bones. Her ebony hair was always pulled into a beehive bun high on her head with chop stick looking ornaments strategically placed to support it. I often wondered what her story was. Where was she from? Assuming she was not a native. How did she come to live in Rochester? What led her to become an apparently successful business woman? This was 1968 or so. Women's liberation hadn't burst into the social consciousness yet. A successful business woman was still a rarity. She walked confidently ahead of us in a fast pace. The pace was as fast as her pattern of speech, my brain raced to catch up with what she said. As she walked, her hips swayed side to side. She wore black, almost stiletto-style heals revealing toe cleavage. She handed us our menus, smiling as we sat down in an intimate corner. I remember one occasion we were at the restaurant and another maître d, attempted to seat us by the kitchen. We knew to request a better table from the fine treatment of the owner.

Cathay Pagoda became our favorite restaurant, not that we experienced plenty of other restaurants. This one was convenient, friendly, the food was good and inexpensive for high school students. After a time, we didn't really need menus. We were familiar enough with the selections. I usually ordered Wonton Soup, with lots of crispy noodles, and either Moo Goo Gai Pan or Moo Sho Chicken. Tea came with the entrée. We were too young for alcoholic beverages, but I would have had sake if given the choice. There was something about how the food was prepared that allowed the distinctive flavor of each ingredient to come through. Even with the addition of sauces as in the case of Moo Goo Gai Pan, you could still taste the individual vegetables—-water chestnuts, peas, mushrooms, baby corn, etc. The sauce just enhanced those flavors. It never over powered them. At that time, I wasn't paying attention to MSG or other food additives. The technique of subtle flavor enhancement using natural ingredients is what interested me most and what I wanted to capture in the Asian inspired stir-fry dish that follows.

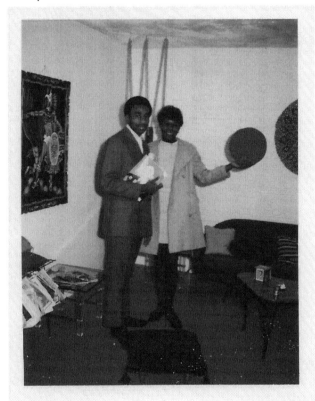

March, 1970 – How we might look going to dinner at Cathay Pagoda

Baby Bok Choy and Mushrooms

Preparation time: 20 minutes
Cooking time: 30 minutes
Serving size: 4

Ingredients:

3 stalks Baby Bok Choy
1 Yellow onion, peeled and sliced
½ lb. Shitake Mushrooms
8 oz. Shrimp, cooked (optional)
1 Tbs. Capers
4 Garlic cloves, sliced

1 Tbs. Olive oil
1 Tbs. Non-dairy butter
1 C. Vegetable stock
1 C. Port Wine
1 Tbs. Black pepper, ground
1 Tbs. Turmeric

Directions:

Rinse the bok choy well. Chop off the bottom ends and separate the leaves from the stem. Set the vegetable aside. Heat olive oil in a sauté pan or wok. Add garlic and stir until fragrant. Add onions and cook until they are translucent. Place mushrooms in the pan and cover the pan. The mushrooms make their own juice. Cook the mushrooms until the juice is absorbed and mushrooms are brown on each side and tender. Add pepper and turmeric followed by butter, vegetable broth and port wine. Place the bok choy in the pan and simmer until the leaves are bright green and tender. If shrimp is added, heat until pink.

Serve:

Place the vegetables in a shallow dish and serve as is or over rice or quinoa.

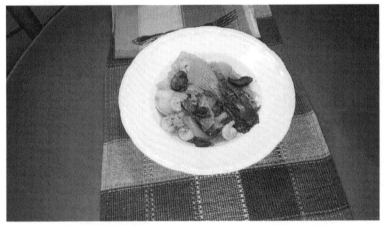

Baby Bok Choy with Mushrooms and Shrimp

Greasy Spoons

My boyfriend and I also liked exploring other types of food and restaurants. We found that some of the best food was at greasy spoons. You know, places where you'd find paper napkins instead of cloth, in fact no table linen at all. There might be sawdust on the floor, a few wait staff without uniforms, and yes maybe a spoon or other cutlery that wasn't gleaming. These establishments concentrated on food preparation and not the aesthetics of the environment.

Nick Tahou's

As a young adult and into my early 20s, I naturally liked to party. Dancing was my thing. I would go anywhere I could dance. Usually it was house parties. Clubs weren't that plentiful in Rochester. If we went to clubs, we'd dance until last call and they kicked us out. We'd either end up at some after-hours joint or at Nick Tahou's.

Nick Tahou's was a diner located on one of the main corridors in Rochester. As most diners do, it had a wide menu selection across each meal from breakfast through dinner. What was unique about Nick Tahou's was its garbage plate menu selection. It became famous for it. While it's not an appetizing sounding name, we found the food in the garbage plate appealing and good. The diner was open 24-hours a day and became the go-to place to satisfy hunger, after a night of partying when the clubs closed. As the story goes, the garbage plate got its name from combining all the unsold food from the day into a serving plate. It usually consisted of hash brown potatoes, hot dog including Rochester's famous white hots, sausages, burgers all covered in Nick's special meat sauce, scrambled eggs, baked beans and maybe a biscuit on the side to sop up all the sauces and juices. It was the meat sauce that made the difference. Of course the meat sauce recipe was a trade secret. However, I'm almost certain it was tomato based. People from all stations and levels in life would find their way to Nick Tahou's.

The place was perfect for people watching. You would find people who make their living from the streets at Nick's—prostitutes all decked out in their working cloths. Mini-skirts, midriff and cleavage revealing halter tops, some kind of feathery or fake fur jacket, if they wore hosiery at all it was fishnet. Platform heals. They were always heavily made up and wig-wearing. Most had cigarettes hanging out the side of their mouth. Their pimps were dressed in the stereotypical way. Three-piece suit, sometimes pen-stripped, colorful shirts and ties with big, thick knots. Platform shoes to match a wide-brimmed hat cocked to one side of his head. Of what you could see of his hair, it was straightened/permed and slicked down. A pimp generally wore an overcoat draped over his shoulders that sort of billowed behind him as he walked. It wasn't surprising to see a pimp and prostitute argue and maybe even fight in Nick's.

While you had the dark side of city life at Nick's, you may also find young white college students, university professors, musicians, other artists and entertainers, young professionals, and all folks in between. One night recently, I had insomnia and in surfing the television shows landed for a time on one of the late night talk shows. The guest being interviewed was comedian Kevin Hart who mentioned being on tour and his next stop was Rochester, NY. The host urged him to go to Nick Tahou's for the garbage plate. It continues to have a long-standing reputation that the famous and anonymous recognize. It was fun to size everyone up and try to guess the relationships of who they were with and their own personal stories. The combination people watching and the food made Nick Tahou's the after-hours place to be. Of course, this is a meal one eats once maybe twice a year. There isn't a single green or fibrous item on the plate. This artery clogging meal is a heart attack waiting to happen.

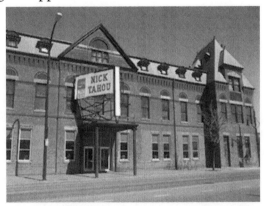

Nick Tahou's, Rochester, NY

The following recipe is a heart healthy answer to the garbage plate using plant-based ingredients on-hand or left-over.

138

Plant-based Garbage Plate

Preparation time: 30 minutes (unless the ingredients are left-overs)
Cooking time: 60 minutes
Serving size: 4

Ingredients:

10 oz. Collard or Southern greens
(mixture of Mustard, Turnip,
Kale, Dandelion)
2 C. Baked Beans (from recipe on
page 119)
1 C. Red or Tri-colored quinoa
5 C. Vegetable broth
3 Tbs. Olive oil

1 Garlic, entire bulb, sliced
1 Onion, yellow, diced
2 C. White potato, cubed
6 Tbs. Garlic Butter
1 Tsp. Black pepper, ground
1 Tbs. Red pepper, crushed
1 Tsp. Nutmeg

Directions:

If you don't already have quinoa on hand, cook quinoa in a 1-quart
sauce pan using 2 cups of vegetable broth and a bit of garlic. Simmer
for about 30 minutes or until all moisture is absorbed and remove
from flame. In a sauté pan heat 1 tablespoon of olive oil and brown
potatoes with 1/4 cup diced onion and a bit of garlic. Season with
black pepper. Place browned potatoes in a dish until ready to serve.

Using a tablespoon of olive oil and garlic butter sauté remaining
onion and garlic until onion is translucent. Add greens and 2 cups
vegetable broth, red pepper and nutmeg and simmer until greens
are tender.

Using remaining garlic butter and vegetable broth make a roux
adding a bit of flour to thicken it slightly.

Serve:

Plate the quinoa topped with greens. Add potatoes and cover it all with the garlic roux. Add baked beans on side. The sweetness of the beans paired with the savory greens, quinoa and potatoes make for a nice flavor contrast in addition to variety of textures..

The Pythod

The Pythod wasn't known for its food. It was known for its music. Jazz specifically. Located on Clarissa Street in the center of Rochester's Black community, The Pythod was a destination location for many up and coming jazz musicians as well as established musicians. The venue itself was a converted single-family house that became a jazz club. There was a main room with a riser as a stage for the musicians. Lighting was arranged to spotlight the stage. I remember seeing there on several occasions, Lonnie Liston Smith as he was known at the time. Dizzie Gillespie, Miles Davis, Wayne Shorter, Terrance Blanchard, Ronnie Laws were among the musicians that played at The Pythod. Because Rochester is situated between Syracuse and Buffalo, musicians found it easy to stop there on their way to and from NYC.

Except for candle-lit table rounds, and the glimmer of a lit cigarette between the fingers of an avid jazz fan, the rest of the room was dark. The audience sipped their drinks, and nodded their heads to the beat of the music listening intently to the likes of Herbie Mann. You didn't go there for the ambience. There was a single stall ladies bathroom and off the main room was a kitchen. The menu was simple— wings, fries, and sandwiches. Not a single fruit or vegetable to be found. There was of course a bar where wine and whiskey was sold. But, you didn't go to The Pythod for the food or drinks. You went for the music. Some of the same people in The Pythod audience, you'd find later at Nick Tahou's or Snuffy's.

Okra Etouffee with Shrimp

Preparation time: 20 minutes
Cooking time: 90 minutes
Serving size: 6-8 servings

Ingredients:

1 lb. Okra
1 Onion, brown – chunked
1 head of garlic, sliced
8 oz. Shishito peppers
1 C. Flour, all-purpose
6 Tbs. Olive oil
4 C. Vegetable broth
4 Tbs. Black pepper, ground
4 Tbs. Red pepper, ground
  (cayenne)

2 lbs. Shrimp, deveined
2 lbs. Crab meat (optional)
1 C. Bourbon (optional) **OR**
1-16 oz. Stewed Tomatoes or
  8 large tomatoes, quartered
  (optional)
Rice or couscous or quinoa

Directions:

In a sauté pan heat 1 tablespoon of olive oil. While the oil is heating, cut ends off of the okra, and slice okra into penny size medallions and set aside. Cut ends off the peppers and set aside. Remove and discard the outer brown layer of the onion and cut into chunks—cut into half, then half again twice. Set the onion aside. Peel and slice the garlic head. Once the pan is heated add the garlic and cook until the slices are toasted. Add onion and cook until translucent you may want to caramelize the onion for added flavor. Sautéing the garlic and onion is an important step not to miss. You don't need to sauté the okra or peppers.

Meanwhile begin making the roux. In a Dutch oven pan heat 5 tablespoons of olive oil. Stir in the flour until it is fully coated with oil. Reduce the flame and continue to stir the mixture until a smooth paste is formed. Allow the flour to brown as you continue to stir the paste to prevent it from sticking to the pan and burning. Add two tablespoons of the seasoning to the roux paste. When it reaches the color you prefer, add the vegetable broth stirring constantly until the liquid has thickened to a silky smooth consistency. Add in the vegetables and remaining seasoning. Let the stew simmer on low heat for 45 minutes. Add the shrimp and or crab and cook until the seafood is pink, and plump about 15 minutes.

During the last 30 minutes of the Etouffee simmering, cook the rice or couscous or quinoa following the directions on the package. I substitute vegetable broth with added minced garlic for water to give it more flavor. Let the rice, couscous or quinoa stand for 5 minutes before serving.

Serve:

Plate the couscous and ladle the Etouffee on top.

NOTE: Because this essentially is a stew (Etouffee is a Cajun word for stew) one would think you could cook all the ingredients in one pot at one time. Don't do it. Sautéing the garlic and onions first, helps to release those flavors. When I first made this dish, I made the mistake of dumping all the vegetables into the roux. I ended up with a bland tasting Etouffee. Those pungent garlic and onion flavors never came through.

Another mistake I made was adding too much flour. More is not always good. A little flour as a thickening agent goes a long way. You want the roux to be just thick enough to cover the bed of rice. Too much was a problem with the peppers too.

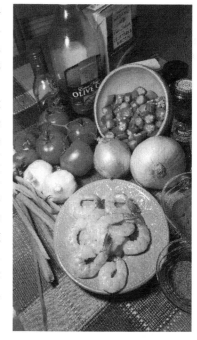

You don't want the dish so spicy it numbs your tongue from tasting the other ingredients. I did that a couple of times. To fix it, in one instance, I added bourbon. In another situation I added stewed tomatoes. In both cases the added ingredients took down the spiciness. Instead of the spice meeting you upon first placing the food in your mouth, it came forward at the end of the bite. It enhanced the dish as it should and didn't overpower it.

Temptations Reunion Tour

Motown was the soundtrack of my life as it was with many of us baby-boomers. My favorite Motown group was and still is the tempting Temptations. In the early 1980s, the group reunited—they were an institution and a sound, no matter who the individuals were that made that sound. Most of the original singers were part of the Reunion Tour—Eddie Kendrick, David Ruffin, Melvin Franklin, Otis Williams and Paul Williams who was deceased by then and replaced. The Tour came to Rochester and oh look out!

My high school girl friends and I went to the concert together as part of a nostalgic experience. We danced in the aisles of the Rochester Armory moving our 34 year old bodies like we were teenagers to The Way You Do the Things You Do, I'm Losing You, My Girl, Ain't Too Proud to beg and other hits. When the show ended about 11 o'clock, we somehow found our way behind the auditorium and watched the Temps jump into a limousine. Now, I generally don't get celebrity star struck. At the time, I was working as a radio and television broadcaster and interviewed personalities and celebrities now and then. I always treated them professionally as I would anyone else. Even now, living in Los Angeles I see celebrities occasionally, but never bother them as they are just going about their lives. I respect and leave them to their privacy. But that night, I became a hollerin', screamin' big-time groupie/stalker.

My friends and I scrambled into a car and quickly followed the limo to the hotel. We found the Temps in the billiard room playing pool. In that moment, I tried to maintain some semblance of dignity and poise and kept my jaw from dropping. I somehow mustered up the nerve to approach them and asked for their autographs. I was able to get Eddie Kendrick's, who I adored, and David Ruffin's signature without swooning into their arms. Oh, what a night. They were polite to us, even though they had performed their butts off and clearly wanted to unwind and be left alone. So we did. We left them to their pool game and headed to Nick Tahou's. I still have their autographs as a reminder of that night. This next recipe has exciting combinations of plant-based ingredients and seasonings that harmonize almost as well as the Temptations.

Fish Fillet Marinara

Preparation time: 15 minutes
Cooking time: 30 minutes
Serving size: 4
This is one recipe inspired by Cajun cooking.

Ingredients:

1 lb. Fish fillet (your choice, cod, halibut, tilapia, etc.) cut into chunks

4 oz. fresh Basil, whole leaves

1 oz. Crimini mushrooms, sliced

1 large yellow onion, sliced

2 Avocados, mashed

1 head Garlic, cloves mashed

2 Tsp. Black pepper, ground

16 oz. Marinara

1 Tbs. Olive oil

½ C. Merlot Wine

Juice of 1 small lemon

Directions:

In a 3-quart sauce pan, toast mushrooms in the olive oil, flipping to brown both sides. Mushrooms make their own flavorful juice. Add garlic, and onion and heat until both the garlic fragrance is released and the onions are translucent. Your kitchen will be filled with a wonderful aroma.

Meanwhile season the fish squeezing fresh lemon juice over both sides, then sprinkle with black pepper. Cut the fillet into chunks. Cut the avocado in half. Stick a knife blade into the avocado pit, pull the pit out. With a spoon, remove the avocado flesh into a bowl and using the spoon mash until the flesh is nearly smooth. A few lumps is fine.

To the mushroom, garlic, and onion mixture add the fish. Cook the fish until edges are brown or the fillet is opaque. Pour in the marinara sauce and wine. Stir until the wine is blended into the sauce.

To thicken the marinara sauce, add the avocado. Let the mixture simmer for about 3 minutes. Stir in basil and heat until you can smell the basil and it becomes wilted. Simmer the mixture for about 10 minutes until the sauce bubbles and fish is flaky.

Serve:

This sauce can be eaten as is or spooned over rice, quinoa or couscous cooked separately.

High School

In those days we had lunch in the High School cafeteria. Underclassman—grades 7 to 10 were required to stay on campus. Upperclassman had the luxury of going off campus for lunch. Lunches were made fresh in the cafeteria kitchens. We usually had a choice of hot lunches like Salisbury steak, mashed potatoes with gravy and green beans or cold lunches like submarine sandwiches. I could take or leave either one, but loved, loved, loved the sticky buns. They were a pastry sprinkled with cinnamon, and chopped walnuts rolled and placed into a muffin pan to bake until golden brown and each bun popped over the top of the pan. Then as they cooled, a glaze of honey was drizzled over them and maybe a dollop of white icing to top it off. It was melt-in-your-mouth wonderful.

High School curriculums in those days included home economics for the girls, wood shop or auto mechanics for the boys. Girls had to learn the basics of housekeeping and did so through home economics. Cooking was part of the lessons. I liked that part. Not only did we get a chance to prepare and cook food—the school was equipped with a working stove and oven, but we ate it too. We were grouped together in teams of 4 to do the cooking. The recipes were never very exotic. I vaguely remember our team cooking a meatloaf made with ground beef. We each had our responsibilities: 1) preparing the oven, 2) assembling utensils and baking dish, 3) preparing the ingredients and seasonings, and 4) mixing everything together for placement in the oven. Although pretty ordinary, this dish had a unique ingredient, or at least one I never associated with meatloaf. It was rolled oats. Not bread crumbs, but dried oatmeal. As strange as it was to us, we mixed in the oatmeal with the ground beef. The mixture was shaped into a loaf in the shallow baking dish and placed in the 350 degree oven for 30 minutes. About half way through cooking, the loaf was topped with ketchup. Surprisingly enough, the oatmeal gave the meatloaf a richer texture without drying it out as you might expect. Combined with the other ingredients and seasonings, it was good.

Today, I replace meatloaf with recipes that feature quinoa or pureed beans like the one that follows.

Acorn Squash, Quinoa & Green Beans

Preparation time: 15 minutes
Cooking time: 45-60 minutes
Serving size: 4

Ingredients:

1 Acorn Squash
1 C. Tri-colored Quinoa
3 C. Vegetable stock
8 oz. Ripe Olives, pitted (sliced or whole)
10 oz. Green beans
½ C. Orange juice

2 Tbs. Garlic, minced
¼ C. Parsley, fresh
2 Tbs. Olive oil
2 Tsp. Nutmeg
1 Tsp. Cinnamon
2 Tbs. Non-dairy butter

Directions:

The squash and quinoa take the longest to cook (about 30 minutes) so start with them first. Heat oven to 350 degrees to roast the squash. Add 2 cups of stock and garlic to taste to 1 cup of quinoa. Bring the mixture to a boil, then turn down the flame to medium low and simmer until all moisture is absorbed. Chop up fresh parsley and add it to the quinoa near the end of cooking time.

Cut the squash length-wise in half. Remove all the seeds and strings. Wash and clean the squash exterior. Coat the outside of the squash with olive oil. Coat the inside of squash with butter. Sprinkle nutmeg and cinnamon on the inside. Place the squash cut side down in a shallow baking dish. Cover the bottom of the dish with orange juice. Place the squash in the heated oven and roast uncovered until fork tender.

In a sauce pan heat remaining vegetable stock, butter and garlic. Stir in green beans and cook until fork tender and bright green. Stir in olives to heat.

Serve:

Slice the squash length-wise after it rests for 5 minutes from the oven. Plate the sliced squash and add a scoop of quinoa alongside green beans and olives.

Boston cream pie and the Diary

I was never one of the cool kids in high school. You probably know the school cafeteria was the location in which the student pecking order was clearly delineated. My two or three girlfriends and I would sit together. In the 9th grade, we were of course all at the same social level. There were three general social level categories—the cool kids, the athletes and the bad kids (kids who were always in trouble-fights, expelled, suspended, etc.). We didn't fit any of those categories. We were an unnamed category of our own—today I'd call us the invisibles. We all tried out for cheerleader. Only one of us made it. She then moved into the category of a cool kid, but continued to run around with us. When I didn't make the cheering squad, I tried out for majorettes. Majorettes marched in parades just ahead of the school band twirling batons, wearing short skirts and boots. Surprisingly enough, I made it. It still didn't make me a cool kid, though. One day while eating Boston cream pie, I decided to write about this strange social segregation.

I was introduced to Boston cream pie by the West High school cafeteria. It had a creamy vanilla pudding filling between two layers of moist yellow cake and topped with rich chocolate icing. I thought it was heaven. These were flavor and texture combinations I had not experienced before. Boston cream pie is actually a cake, why it's called a pie, I don't know. I also don't know for sure what about that dessert made me think of writing about this segregation of students. Maybe it was the different layers of the "pie" that I equated with the different student social categories.

Homeroom was a quiet period during the school day where students are expected to study, or do homework. Bored with homework and studying, I used my homeroom period to write, like in a diary, about the athletes, specifically the football players who choose to follow this informal practice of excluding anyone who was outside of their athletic world from even common courtesies like saying hello. They walked around like they ruled. If you dared speak to them, they were not likely to respond as you weren't worthy of their attention. Many of them were in my homeroom. They only acknowledged their team mates, cheerleaders, and one English teacher. Miss R. She was young and good looking. She dressed well in form fitting dresses and skirts revealing a well-proportioned figure. It was rumored she was having an affair with one of the football players. I never mentioned it in my writing; however, I did name all who acted "stuck up." I wrote about how they were so taken with themselves, describing their behavior, physiques, and assigning nicknames that matched their personalities or what I thought of them. At some point the team quarterback began paying attention to me and started teasing me. He acted totally out of character for an athlete and blurred the lines of what was the socially accepted high school structure. When I didn't respond thinking he was just being mean, he snatched away my diary with descriptions of the football team and began reading it. He laughed as he walked away with it taunting me. The next homeroom period was very different. The athletes I wrote about all said hello to me as they passed my desk. I was stunned and embarrassed. The quarterback apparently shared the diary with his teammates and I became the homeroom class joke. It was humiliating.

Tommy's Grocery Store

Food was even connected to where we lived in the early days. When we came to live with my uncle and his wife in the early 1960s, we lived in a two-bedroom apartment over the neighborhood grocery store—Tommy's. Couldn't get any closer to food than that. Home gardening was passé at that time and for us there wasn't any room for it. Community gardens were unheard of. Tommy's would supplement our food supply between supermarket shopping. Chiefly when we ran out of eggs, bread, milk and sugar, we'd run down to Tommy's. Tommy's was owned by Tommy and his wife Peggy. They were one of the few remaining white couples in the neighborhood. Don't know what their ethnicity was. Can't remember their last names. They worked long hours keeping that corner store going. It was a staple for our family in a crunch. It sat right on the southwest corner of Magnolia and Plymouth. There was parking in the back, but everyone who shopped at Tommy's was within walking distance. Tenants in the three apartments above used the lot to park their cars, if they had them.

I remember seeing Peggy walking to work to fill her shift. She always wore slacks. Usually black with a cotton blouse. I don't remember ever seeing her in a dress or skirt. She was about 5' 7". Slender. Blonde. I don't think it was natural. She was never without makeup. In fact, Peggy was heavily made up every time I saw her. Blue eye shadow, black eyeliner and mascara, her eyebrows were penciled in and arched high. Her lipstick was bright red and just outside her lip line. She wore black rimmed glasses. Nails were well polished. Her shoes were like nurses shoes because she had to be on her feet all day. She sometimes wore espadrilles and changed them once she was behind the store counter. Her walk was almost runway like. One foot directly in front of the other that caused her hips to sway a bit. She had perfect posture.

Behind the counter, Peggy was a chain smoker and always had a cigarette lit. It was either dangling from her mouth or burning in a nearby ashtray. Depending on the time of day, Peggy would have the television on watching her soaps while she worked. She spoke with a raspy, husky voice. I'm sure it was from her smoking. I remember her having a dry sense of humor. Her demeanor was low-key friendly, respectful but distant without much warmth. I always felt that Peggy had her sights set on more in life, but she settled. I don't believe the couple had any children. If they did, the children weren't part of the business and never came around.

Tommy was a soft spoken guy with a slight accent of some sort. He was ordinary looking with gray hair and a receding hair line. Tommy was slender and slightly shorter than Peggy. He wore specs as well. He always wore a full apron when he worked behind the counter, which I found interesting since he didn't supply fresh meat like a butcher. When his wife worked, she never wore an apron. Tommy's apron covered khaki slacks and blue button down shirts. It became kind of his work uniform. Tommy seemed to have a bit more energy than Peggy. He was taking inventory, or stocking shelves or otherwise multi-tasking while working the counter. Peggy just worked the counter. Yet she supported him and the business. They were very much a couple and business partners. That came across in the rare moments when they were seen together—during shift changes.

In the summer of 1964 when I was thirteen, Rochester's Black community erupted across town on the north side of the city. Ironically, in the land that slavery abolitionist Fredrick Douglas and woman's suffragette Susan B. Anthony found sanctuary and made their homes a century earlier, generated rising discontent in the Black community of the 1960s that finally boiled over. A white police officer pulled over a car driven by a Black driver and passenger, allegedly for a burned out tail light. The stop escalated into one of the first riots of that period. The Watts riots hadn't yet happened. The incident ignited a pot of simmering, seething grievances of injustices long suffered by the Black community without recourse or outlet for constructive expression.

While most of the uprising took place across town, there were outbreak pockets that surfaced on the west side where there were neighborhoods populated with high concentrations of African Americans. However, it never reached the south west side of the city where we lived. By day three, I vividly remember watching as the National Guard in their camouflage tanks and jeeps rolled down Plymouth Avenue from our balcony over Tommy's store. I remember thinking how significant that was. Enraged Black people unleashed the only power they had that couldn't be contained by the local police department. Governor Rockefeller had to send the army and National Guard to control the power. The entire City was on lockdown for at least 5 days after the riot started, with nightly curfews. The air was thick with tension. Through it all, Tommy's Grocery was never attacked and remained open. Tommy and Peggy took the risk to keep the store going. Although with limited hours, they were available for us and any neighbor who cared to venture out to get food. We could feel the anxiety from the adults. For me and some of the kids there was a nervous excitement. During this time, we abandoned our usual weekly menu selections for more casual, and comfortable fare like Sloppy Joes. The following recipe is a simple plant-based Sloppy Joes.

Sloppy Joes for Vegans

Preparation time: 15 minutes
Cooking time: 20 minutes
Serving size: 4

Ingredients:

4 Tbs. Olive Oil, extra virgin
1 Garlic head, chopped
¼ C. Green onion
¼ C. Chives, Chopped
1 Yellow Onion, chopped
1 Green bell pepper, diced
1 C. Red Kidney beans (soaked, drained)

1 Tsp Black pepper, ground
2 Tsp. Cumin
¼ Tsp. Coriander
¼ C. Brown Sugar
16 oz. Tomato sauce
4 Round buns, pre-sliced

Directions:

In a medium sauce pan pour 1 Tbs. of olive oil and heat with low flame. To the heated oil add bell pepper, onions (yellow and green), and garlic. Allow them to become tender and the released flavors to mingle. Stir the vegetables and add the seasonings pepper, cumin, coriander. Allow them to mix for 5 to 8 minutes more stirring constantly. As you know by now the beans can be soaked overnight or at least 5 hours prior to using. Drain the soaked beans. They can then be processed in a food processor. They should have a rough texture, not a paste. They are then ready to be added to the sautéed vegetables and spices mixture to cook.

Add the roughly mashed kidney beans and mix until the beans are fully blended with the vegetables and spices. If the mixture begins to stick while heating, add a splash of vegetable broth to loosen the ingredients. Once the broth cooks off, stir in the tomato sauce and brown sugar. Let the mixture simmer about 20 minutes more or until all the ingredients have become incorporated into the sauce.

Serve:

Spoon the sloppy joes sauce over 1/2 of a toast bun, place the other 1/2 bun on top and serve.

Seafood Crepe

Preparation time: 10 minutes
Cooking time: 30 minutes
Serving size: 4

Ingredients:

½ C. Flour
⅛ C. Almond Milk
¼ C. Egg whites
4 Tbs. Olive Oil
1 Garlic head, chopped
¼ C. Green onion
¼ C. Chives, Chopped

½ C. Crimini mushrooms, sliced
½ lb. Fish fillet chunked (cod, cat fish, white fish)
¼ lb. Shrimp
2 Tsp. Black pepper
2 Tsp. Cumin
½ C. White wine

Directions:

Crepe sauce – In a sauce pan heat olive oil. Add garlic, green onion, and chives. Cook until garlic is slightly brown, the onion and chives are fragrant. Add mushrooms to the mixture. Your kitchen will come alive with the wonderful aromas of garlic, onion, chives and mushrooms harmonizing like a well- rehearsed Baptist church choir.

While that magic is happening, season the fish with cumin and black pepper. Add the fish to the sauce pan of vegetables followed by the shrimp. Actually, you can use the seafood of your choice. What shows in the recipe are my preferences. I'd stay away from fish fillets that easily break up when cooked. Allow the seafood to cook with the vegetables until the fish are flaky or in the case of shrimp, they're pink. Over a medium flame, slowly stir in flour to the pan of juices created by both the vegetables and fish. The flour will begin to clump. When that happens add a splash or two of almond milk. Stirring constantly, pour in the wine until the clumped flour breaks down and becomes a creamy sauce of medium thickness or the thickness of your liking. Simmer the mixture until creamy but continue stirring to avoid the roux sticking to the bottom of the pan.

Pancake – In a bowl, mix egg white, and milk with pancake batter. Add enough milk to make a thin batter. In a sauté pan with heated olive oil, pour the batter to make a thin pancake. When the edges begin to curl and are lightly brown, turn the pancake to brown on the other side—about 3 minutes each side. When lightly browned, remove the pancake to a dish. The pancake should be pliable.

Serve:

Place the thin pancake on a plate. Pour the seafood sauce down the middle of the pancake. Fold the sides of the pancake into the middle with the ends open. Ladle more sauce over the top and serve. Umm, is that good! Although there's flour used to make the sauce and a pancake base, the dish is surprisingly light.

Pets & Food

Feifei was our pet Chihuahua. Why the French name Feifei for a Mexican Chihuahua, I don't know. It must have been an inside joke. Or maybe my mother didn't know any better. Feifei was one of my early memories. She was a fierce little thing. Very protective of me and my sister. When anyone approached us that she didn't know, her ears would perk up, she'd bare her teeth and growl, then bark ferociously at them until they backed away. You couldn't come near us with Feifei on the scene.

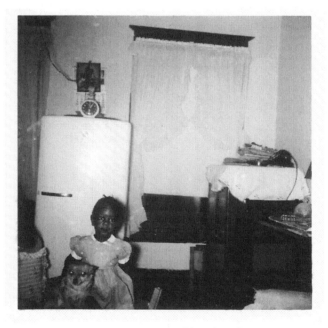

Me at 2 or 3 years old and Feifei

When we moved from Stillson Street to St. Claire, Feifei came with us. I felt secure in our new place knowing Feifei would warn us of any danger as we got used to our new home. But shortly after our move, Feifei was stolen. We were heart-broken. After a time, we got a new dog, Peanuts. It was a mixture Basset hound and dachshund. He was nothing like Feifei in temperament and disposition. Peanuts was much friendlier. He wasn't a protector, but more of a playmate. He was laid back and indifferent about strangers approaching us. He did have one aggressive trait—that of chasing cars. Whenever a car came down our end of the street, Peanuts would chase after it barking. I didn't understand why he did that or what he would do if he caught up with the car. I preferred the fearlessness of Feifei. Unfortunately, Peanuts wasn't with us long. A car he was chasing ran him over.

With all of our pets, I don't remember them being fed dog food. Dog food wasn't as promoted and used as much as it is today—especially today's trend toward healthy dog food. I find it ironic that some pet owners (I'm sure not any of you) pay more attention to what they feed their dogs than what they themselves eat. Dogs in particular have been eating out of garbage bins and drinking out of toilets forever. Now pampered pets eat better than some humans. But I digress. Our pets ate the same food we did. It was our scrapes, but the same food nonetheless. We were careful not to feed them any bones that would splinter or chocolate, even before we knew how harmful those items were to dogs. We figured, if it's good enough for us, it's good enough for our pet dog.

With Peanuts death, I was unable to invest my feelings into another pet. After mother's death when we lived with our uncle and his wife, they got a dog and named it Dusty. I never grew close to Dusty. I haven't had any pets since. When he was about 8 or 9, my son wanted a dog. He got goldfish instead.

Shrimp & Grits

Preparation time: 5 minutes
Cooking time: 20 minutes
Serving size: 4

Ingredients:

¾ C. Grits
1 lb. Shrimp, frozen, peeled
3 Tbs. Garlic, heaping
4 Chive sprigs, chopped
½ Onion, Yellow

1½ Avocado
1 Tbs. Cayenne pepper
2 Tbs. Turmeric
1 Tbs. Non-dairy butter
1½ C. Vegetable stock

This is one of those dishes that may be served as a breakfast.

Directions:

Roux: In a sauté pan melt butter, then add onion, and chives and sauté until translucent. Add a splash of vegetable broth and remove the mixture from heat.

Grits: Place remaining vegetable broth in a medium sauce pan, stir in 2 tablespoons of minced garlic and bring it to a boil. Slowly stir in grits. Continue to stir grits until they begin to thicken. The vegetable broth will turn the grits a warm brown color. To give the grits a creamy consistency without using dairy products, add mashed avocados with remaining garlic. Blend in the turmeric and cayenne. Just enough cayenne to give it a kick. A little goes a long way. Between the seasonings and avocado, the grits will take on the color of the avocado. Fold in the onion & chives to the mixture. As the grits begin to bubble add the shrimp. There should be enough shrimp to have with each spoonful of grits. Let the pan simmer for 5 minutes. To thin the grits add a splash or two more vegetable broth. To thicken, allow the liquid to cook down. You'll have to constantly stir the pot to keep the grits from sticking.

Serve:

Ladle the shrimp and grits into a shallow bowl and serve with biscuits.

86 Meigs Street & Culinary Curiosity

It was the address of my first apartment and the place that became my cooking laboratory. Meigs Street was located in the artsy, bohemian section of my hometown, Rochester. It was 1971. I was 20 years old and finished or about to finish Monroe Community College. Meigs Street was off Park Avenue. Just as the Park Avenue name connotes, the neighborhood aspired to be upscale, but wasn't quite, yet. Yuppies were beginning to come into vogue and move into the area. Yuppies was the nickname given to Young Urban Professionals. I didn't consider myself a Yuppie. At the time, I was still trying to figure myself out. Meigs Street was part of a walking neighborhood, like much of Rochester. You could walk to the Parkleigh pharmacy to buy everything from cookbooks and stationary to body oils and incense to pharmaceuticals. You could walk to Wegman's supermarket for groceries and just about everything else. There were boutique shops selling unique items like hand-crafted jewelry or needlework and bookstores were scattered about the neighborhood. The neighborhood was full of huge two and three story Victorian–style houses many of them converted into apartments. 86 Meigs Street was one of those.

My apartment was located in the rear of the house. It was a 1-bedroom completely furnished apartment. I used to joke when friends came over for the first time. You could stand in the middle of the room and tour the entire place. You'd see the kitchen, living, and bedroom standing in one spot. There was an open closet you entered from the bedroom to reach the bathroom. The closet joined the two rooms. I moved there because the rent was affordable, furniture was supplied, and I felt safe even though you entered from the rear. There were plenty of flood lights to light the way to my door when it got dark. When I was home, besides the bedroom, I spent most of my time in the kitchen experimenting with recipes.

It was a galley kitchen. There was no room to sit. A counter top on the left side, porcelain sink at the end with corner shelving on either side of the sink to hold plants or other decorative pieces. On the right was the apartment-sized stove next to an apartment-sized refrigerator. Above the stove was cabinet space to store dishes, canned goods, spices. Below the sink was space for pots and pans, cleaning products and a trash can. That was my kitchen.

I love to cook. It stimulates creativity in me. It's relaxing and gratifying especially when a dish turns out right in taste and presentation and those you cook for express their enjoyment. For me, the act of cooking is somehow therapeutic. Now with my own kitchen, I could create and experiment until I got tired. Eager to learn new dishes, I perfected lasagna, learned to make eggplant parmesan, zucchini and pumpkin breads, and cooked my first duck.

Cooking duck was an experience. I had gotten a recipe from one of my library of cookbooks. The recipe seemed simple enough. I bought a small duck, maybe about 3 pounds, after all it was just me who would be the guinea pig before experimenting with my friends. I prepared it as the recipe instructed with seasoning. Placed it on a rack in a shallow roasting pan in a pre-heated oven at 325 degrees. As it cooked the smell of the seasonings began to take over the apartment. It smelled wonderful. Checking on the bird, after a time, I noticed the amount of grease that was cooking out of it. It was enough to nearly fill the shallow roasting pan. No need to baste this bird. I emptied the drippings into an empty orange juice carton and put the duck back into the oven to continue roasting.

I must have performed that same routine about 4 different times and the grease kept coming. I ran out of containers to put the grease in. I heard and read that ducks had a lot of fat, but I had no idea. It just didn't end. I grew concerned that the meat would be tough, because by now the duck had roasted for about 5 hours, at least two hours over what the recipe called for. The skin was more charred than crispy. The duck had shrunk down to nothing. Finally, I took the shriveled bird out of the oven. Let it "rest" for about 30 minutes. I carved a piece to taste and was overwhelmed by the grease. It took over any flavor. I was crushed my roast duck didn't turn out like I had hoped but grateful there were no witnesses to this disaster. I hate throwing away food, especially meat, even in my early days of experimentation. Meat is too expensive. After all … there are starving children in Africa. I'd always find a use for unsuccessful dishes, but this was unsalvageable. I threw away the duck, as far away as I could. It was too horrible for human consumption. Could have given it to a dog I suppose, but dogs weren't allowed in the building. Besides, I have a feeling even a dog would have rejected it.

This next recipe is a lot less complicated than roast duck.

Broccoli and Quinoa

Preparation time: 10 minutes
Cooking time: 30 minutes
Serving size: 4

Ingredients:

8 oz. Broccoli

4 oz. Crimini Mushrooms

1 C. Tri-colored, Quinoa

3 C. Vegetable broth

1 Tbs. Olive oil

1 Garlic, entire bulb, sliced

Onion, yellow, minced

½ C. Pine nuts

¼ C. Garlic Butter

1 Tsp. black pepper, ground

Directions:

In a small sauce pan bring 2 cups of vegetable broth to a boil. Add quinoa and stir. Reduce the flame to low and let the quinoa simmer until all the moisture is absorbed. When the moisture is absorbed, remove the quinoa from the heat and let it stand.

In a sauté pan heat the olive oil, then add onion, mushrooms, and garlic. When the onion becomes translucent add pine nuts to toast them. The pine nuts gives this dish a bit more crunch and texture. Once the pine nuts are toasted add the broccoli and garlic butter. Stir the combination until the broccoli is a bright green and a bit crunchy. Stir in the quinoa and black pepper until thoroughly mixed.

Plate the dish and serve immediately.

Chevy Impala

I graduated high school in 1969— the year of the most stylish Ford Cougar, in my opinion. I loved that car mostly because of the way the turn signal displayed. You'd see a light sequence of red from left to right or right to left depending on the direction you wanted to turn. It was the coolest look to me. I was fond of the yellow color, appropriate for a Cougar. It reminded me of the animal. My uncle was afraid I'd run off with the first guy who drove up in a Cougar. I promised I wouldn't, but if a guy came calling in a yellow Cougar, who knows what I might have done. When I saved up enough money to buy a car, it was neither new or a 1969 Ford Cougar. It was a 1957 Chevy Impala.

A tank of a car. It was a faded sky blue color with rust spots from the salt used in Rochester's attempt to guard against icy roads during harsh winters. I bought it from an acquaintance of a co-worker. The interior was in relatively good shape. It ran well although loud. You could hear it coming a mile away. It served me well during the time that I had it. It got me off dependency from public transportation and friends to go back and forth to work and school. It was the car my youngest sister, Barbara, used to help get her learner's permit, then her driver's license.

My boyfriend at the time didn't own a car and had to borrow from friends. When I bought my car I thought we could use it to go to drive-in movies. I used to love going to the Empire Drive-In in Webster when I was little with my Mother, her friend, and my sister. We'd be dressed in our pajamas. Don't remember the films as much as I remember the food. Drive-in movie food was always good. There were burgers, dogs, and French fries, cracker jacks, and popcorn. Somehow the burgers, fries and dogs tasted better at the drive-in. Maybe it was the fresh air.

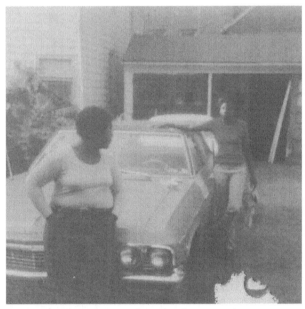

Barbara in front, me on the side of my Impala –Aug. 1974

Don & Bob's

When the subject of burgers comes up, usually Don & Bob's is part of the conversation. Don & Bob's was a burger joint in the suburb of Irondequoit situated on the bay. It earned a reputation for some of the biggest and best tasting burgers in town. The burgers were made large enough to spill over the bun. They were loaded with chopped onion, pickle relish and some kind of ketchup and mustard combination that kicked up the flavor. Don & Bob's was only open during the summer months. While these foods are no longer part of my life, they illustrate the significant role they played in my early years.

Instead of burgers, I now eat sandwiches like the Panini in the following recipe.

Quinoa, Red Onion, Avocado Panini

Preparation time: 20 minutes
Cooking time: 30 minutes
Serving size: 4

Ingredients:

1 C. Quinoa, tri-colored
2 C. Vegetable stock, organic low-sodium
4 Tbs. Garlic, minced
2 Avocados, ripened

¼ C. Red Onion, diced
½ C. Sugar Plum Tomatoes, cut in half
2 Tsp. Horseradish
4 Panini bread pieces, toasted

Directions:

In a 1-quart sauce pan pour vegetable broth and bring to a boil over high flame. Add the quinoa and 2 heaping tablespoons of minced garlic and stir. When the mixture comes to a boil, reduce the flame to low and simmer until all the liquid is absorbed by the quinoa about 30 minutes. Remove the quinoa from the flame and let it cool down.

While the quinoa is simmering, dice the red onion and split the tomatoes in half placing both ingredients in a medium-size bowl. Cut and scoop the avocados from their shell into a small mixing bowl. Using a potato masher, mash the avocados for a smooth consistency. Add 2 tablespoons of minced garlic and 2 teaspoons of horseradish for a light kick. Mix these ingredients and let stand until the quinoa has cooled down.

Place the cooled quinoa in a large mixing bowl. Blend in the red onion and tomatoes. Add the avocado mixture to the bowl ingredients and stir thoroughly until the avocado completely coats the quinoa mixture. Place the bowl ingredients in the refrigerator at least 1 hour. When ready to serve, toast the Panini bread. Spread the avocado/quinoa mixture on the toasted bread

McCurdy's Tea Room

I have worked since I was 14. One of my early jobs was as a switchboard operator at McCurdy's one of the major downtown department stores in Rochester. Back in the day, incoming calls were connected to the proper department through a third party mechanism operated by a person. That was me and my five colleagues. When a call came into McCurdy's on one of several phone lines, we'd answer and through our headset ask to what department the caller wished to be connected. With a cord that corresponded to the incoming call, we'd connect the caller to their party. It was fun in the beginning. After a while it became monotonous. You'd have to find ways to keep it interesting. I was grateful for the job, but glad I worked there part-time after school and on weekends only. I earned money to buy my school clothes. As an employee, I'd get the store discount. What I didn't spend on clothes, I'd save to buy books for classes at MCC and towards a car. On weekends, when I worked a full day, I'd take lunch in the restaurant located in the store's basement. The Tea Room.

The Tea Room was decorated to simulate an English garden where ladies could go to have their afternoon tea. A white lattice trellis lined the walls with ivy made of silk flower material interlaced between the lattices. White pillars placed in the center gave the large open room some architectural interest. There were no windows in this basement restaurant. However, it was always brightly lit with overhead florescent lights. Round tables covered in white table linen and elaborately folded cloth napkins filled the room. At the entrance to the room was a maître d's station where you checked in to be seated. They'd sometimes take reservations for special events like a fashion show happening at the Tea Room. At one end of the room was a wall covered in a floral wallpaper. I always felt the room was decorated by someone's grandmother.

The restaurant was usually filled with women past their prime who still dressed formally with hats and gloves to go shopping downtown. They seemed to love the McCurdy's Tea Room setting. I came there for the convenience. It didn't happen often, but occasionally I'd have lunch with my middle sister Diane who also worked at McCurdy's on the sales floor. Our hours rarely seemed to match.

On the menu you would find items like Bacon, Lettuce, and Tomato (BLT) sandwiches, Club sandwiches, lady finger cucumber or cream cheese sandwiches without crusts, Spinach Salad, Garden Salad, and for dessert, Boston cream pie or Strawberry Shortcake. My usual was a Turkey Club. It came with pickles and potato chips. I drank either iced tea or lemonade with the sandwich. This is a good illustration of how much more sophisticated our food preferences have become over time, personally and as a society. Today, the Tea Room might be renamed some sort of Bistro. Its menu might include roasted red bell pepper, eggplant, and Portobello mushroom sandwich on focaccia bread with kale chips.

Roasted Bell Pepper, Eggplant & Portobello Sandwich

Preparation time: 20 minutes
Cooking time: 20 minutes
Serving size: 2

Ingredients:

2 Red Bell Peppers, whole
1 Eggplant, sliced into medallions
1 Portobello mushroom, whole
2 Avocados

2 Tbs. Non-dairy butter
4 Tbs. Garlic, minced
5 Tbs. Italian salad dressing
4 Focaccia bread pieces, toasted

Directions:

Coat the bell peppers, eggplant and Portobello with the Italian salad dressing. If the Portobello is too thick, you may slice it for ease in managing it in the sandwich. Roast the bell peppers over a gas range flame until blackened. Remove the blackened skin and set the tender bell pepper aside. Grill the eggplant and Portobello until tender. Spread the focaccia bread with butter and garlic and toast. Mash the avocado in its casing and spread onto two pieces of the bread. Layer the bell pepper, eggplant, Portobello on top of the avocado. Drizzle remaining salad dressing on the vegetable layer and top with the remaining bread.

This is such a hefty sandwich made so by the Portobello, avocados, and the bread. You'll be thoroughly satisfied and wonder why you haven't tried this before.

Serve:

Cut the sandwiches in half and serve with garlic flavored kale chips, shoestring sliced carrots, or celery. These sides are of course optional.

Restaurant Surfing

When I worked in Rochester broadcasting in the 1980s, Trey, the station's promotions assistant, and I became good friends within a few months of his hiring. Trey is this slender, white guy who never gained any weight no matter how much he ate. He's average height with a large appetite for fine food. Trey was energetic with an outgoing personality. He was an aspiring performer—stage, musical theater in particular. Rochester broadcasting was just a stepping stone. Trey has an easy laugh. We used to crack each other up over the silly situations people found themselves in, their idiosyncrasies, or our own simple risk taking. Things we would do just to see how far we could go without getting caught. I remember us crashing an exclusive evening promotional event.

There was plenty of high quality food at the event and the affair was filled to capacity. We used the name of a lifestyle personality we knew was on the guest list and was supposed to attend. Trey confidently dropped the name of the personality to gain entry into the party. Without any further questioning or drama, we were both invited in. As party crashers do, we walked in like we were supposed to be there. Trey and I'd lunch together nearly every day discovering new restaurants or exploring different types of cuisine. I was easily bored with the same old things and always open to trying something new and different especially when it came to food. It was great fun. We tried most restaurants within walking distance from the station. When we dined at all the worthy nearby spots, we eventually ventured out of the neighborhood to places we needed to travel by car.

Rochester was considered (probably still is) a mid-size city with a population at the time of just under one million in the Greater Rochester area. Nevertheless, there was a cultural mix not usually seen by metropolises of its size. A range of racial and ethnic groups were attracted by companies like Eastman Kodak, Xerox, Bausch & Lomb, General Motors and universities like the University of Rochester, Rochester Institute of Technology and St. John Fisher College. There were Asians including Chinese, Japanese, East Indian, and towards the end of my time in Rochester a great influx of Vietnamese and Cambodians. There were Latinos largely from Puerto Rico, some Cubans, and Portuguese. The people of African descent consisted of Jamaican, Nigerian, and of course African-American. Historically there were neighborhoods with people of Irish, Jewish, Polish, German and Italian descent.

Naturally, with this assortment of people comes a variety of cuisine. Not all of the cultures were represented in the restaurant scene though, but enough to offer a variety of food choices. During this time I noticed similarities in food between different cultures. It seems nearly every cultural cuisine has a dish composed of some ingredient stuffed with a filling. egg rolls, Moo Shu chicken (Asian); burritos, taquitos (Latin); po' boys (Southern, African American); Manicotti (Italian), you get the idea. Most cultures have meat at the center of their dishes, except Middle Eastern food. I realized my affinity to Middle Eastern food through restaurant surfing. Without relying on meat, Middle Eastern food is flavorful, relatively light, but filling, and I feel good after eating it. The following recipe is inspired by Middle Eastern cuisine.

Curried Yellow Squash, Zucchini and Garbanzo Beans

Preparation time: 10 minutes
Cooking time: 20 minutes
Serving size: 2

Ingredients:

2 Yellow squash, sliced ¼" thick medallions
1 Zucchini squash, sliced ¼" medallions (optional)
1 Brown onion sliced
1 C. Garbanzo beans, dry, then soaked & cooked

1 Tbs. Olive Oil
¼ C. Vegetable broth
2 Tbs. Garlic, minced
3 Tbs. Curry powder
½ Tsp. Turmeric, ground

Directions:

The garbanzo beans should be soaked and pre-cooked using the instructions in a previous section of this book.

After removing the brown outer covering of the onion, slice it in half length-wise. With the flat half turned down on the cutting board, cut the onion in thin slices across the width. Pour olive oil in a 10" sauté pan to heat over low flame. Add onion and cook until caramelized. For those of you unfamiliar with the technique of caramelization, it is cooking the onion until most of it is brown and a bit crispy. It releases a sweet flavor. But don't worry, the other spices and vegetables tempers the sweetness with savory to give this dish a proper balance. Spoon in garlic and stir. Add the squash. Stir in the curry powder and turmeric. Increase the flame to medium. Sauté until the squash is tender. The squash will generate its own broth during cooking. About 5 minutes before the squash is tender, add the garbanzo beans. I doubt you will need it, but just in case you need more liquid add a splash of the vegetable broth.

Serve:

Hot on dinner plate.

Grunion Run – Malibu

Restaurant surfing, and party crashing were among the many adventures Trey and I experienced. The two of us ended up moving to the West Coast separately within three years of each other. He came first and three years later I followed. Although we were friends and hung out a lot together, we were never a couple. Not only is he 10 years younger, and although we love each other dearly, we are not attracted to each other in that way. He and I are both attracted to men. We ended up in Los Angeles where our adventures continued. One excursion was a trip to witness a Grunion run in Malibu.

Grunions are a type of fish, small to medium sized that use high tide to wash up on the beach where they burrow into the sand to lay eggs. This is an annual occurrence during spring, usually only a two-week window sometime in March when the moon is full and tides are, of course, high. Trey and I, voyeurs that we are, vowed to experience this phenomenon.

One evening in March, we met for dinner at a Malibu restaurant that sits on the beach. Naturally, it has ocean facing windows. We sat at a table with full view of the beach and could watch the sunset. We had a lovely seafood dinner, wine, and conversation. When it grew dark, we kept our eye on the beach for Grunion sightings. Over dessert, we spotted a school of Grunions just washed up on the shore. We hurriedly finished dessert and made our way to the beach. We were going to be part of a naturally occurring ritual specific to this region of the country. How exciting. I was eager to become a witness.

Between the restaurant and the beach were rock breakers that decreased from boulders to rocks to stones that became pebbles as you got closer to shore. We had to walk through these to reach the shoreline. Although we knew we'd be Grunion watching, we were still dressed in more than casual wear appropriate to the restaurant's ambiance. To make our way to the beach we removed our shoes. I wore cute little sandals with my sundress. Trey rolled up his pant legs. We plotted our way to the shoreline. With only moonlight and the scant light from the restaurant, we climbed up one rock and down another in the darkness. Trey helped me navigate the rocks. At one point I slipped and cut my leg. I could feel the blood running down my shin. Scraped shin or not, we were determined to see this rare fish ritual. Finally, with a bleeding shin and sore feet, we reached the shoreline. But ... ah ... where are the Grunions?

We were in the spot we saw schools of them from the restaurant window, but they were not there. The tide came in several times as we were stumbling our way to the spot so there should be hundreds of these little creatures, burrowing away. Finally, we realized that what we actually saw were pebbles that appeared to be moving as the tide retreated. There were no Grunions, nowhere. It must've been the wine. All I took away from that little excursion was a cut shin and an amusing memory.

Cajun Fish

Preparation time: 30 minutes
Cooking time: 60 minutes
Serving size: 4-6

Ingredients:

2 Tbs. Olive oil
6 Green onions, medallion sliced
1 Head of Garlic, sliced
4 Tbs. Black pepper
25 oz. Tomato or marinara sauce
⅛ C. dry Red Wine (merlot)

⅛ C. Flour
3 Fish fillet (cod, halibut, haddock) cut into chunks
1 small lemon, juice
2 Tbs. Cayenne or red pepper

Directions:

This is a one pot meal. In a Dutch oven pan heat olive oil and add green onions and garlic. Heat until the onions are tender. Season the fish fillet with lemon juice and black pepper. To the pan, add seasoned fish fillet chunks. Cook until the fish is opaque. Add red pepper and tomato sauce. Stir in flour until it is smooth and allow the sauce to thicken. To the mixture add the red wine. Simmer the ingredients for 15 minutes and the fish is flaky. Remove from heat and let it stand for 5 minutes before serving.

Serve:

Ladle the Cajun fish into a shallow bowl and serve with cornbread.

Bowling & Michael T.

At some point, the two girlfriends I hung out with decided I needed a boyfriend. After all at 13, they each had a guy they were "going with." It hadn't really crossed my mind and wouldn't for a couple of years yet. They arranged a group "date" at a bowling alley.

We all knew Michael since elementary school. His skin was caramel colored with curly black hair and skinny. He walked on his toes. He wore black-rimmed glasses. He was the smartest guy in our class. A title he retained all the way through high school. He was quite nerdy. As nerds are, he was awkward in social situations. We all knew Michael would someday become a doctor. I heard later that destiny was fulfilled. Why my friends thought we'd make a good couple, I'll never know. I didn't consider myself nerdy or as smart as Michael. I was shy but if I had to, I could hold my own in social situations.

We were all too young to drive. I walked to one of my friend's house and together we were driven to the bowling alley. I didn't know or suspect boys would be there. If my uncle and aunt had known, I probably wouldn't have been allowed to go. Shoot, had I known, I probably wouldn't have shown up. So here I am at the bowling alley with my two girlfriends, their boyfriends and Michael. Michael??!! What's he doing here?! I'm sure my friends thought they were doing me a big favor. I felt ambushed, but tried to make the best of it. We were in a group situation, it wasn't like we were paired up. But we were. Michael wasn't bad looking, he just wasn't my type. What was my type at 13? I have no idea what he thought of me. I wondered did he know about the set-up or was he ambushed too?

I don't remember what I wore, but I certainly wasn't dressed to impress. Then there were those horrible looking bowling shoes. You know, the two-toned oxford kind that has your shoe size labeled on the back. How awful!! It wouldn't have been so bad had my shoe size been a dainty size 6, but I wore a size 9. Way too big for a girl my age. They looked like clown shoes on me. My friends, who were my age, wore size 7. I had never bowled before that day and had to learn. Lots of stuff to overcome for a 13 year old. I tried to have fun and relax. I paid attention to how my friends picked out their bowling ball. Tried to understand how to hold the ball and ball placement to knock all the pins down. I learned that when you knock down all the pins with one blow of the ball it's called a strike. The more strikes, the better for you. How hard can that be? I determined if nothing else, at least I was going to bowl well.

It was my turn again. After previously throwing gutter balls, I would take my time and aim differently. I picked up my ball, held it in front of me both elbows bent down with one hand holding the ball, the other bracing it as I eyed where in the alley I wanted the ball to land to hit a strike. Just as I had seen my friends do. Once I pinpointed the spot, I swung back my arm with the ball. As I did, the ball left my fingers, dropped onto the floor and rolled backwards, in what seemed like slow motion, until it rolled off the bowling platform. My friends, Michael, and the entire bowling hall howled in laughter. It was a nightmare. I was mortified. I wanted the floor to open up and swallow me whole. After that moment, my memory is fuzzy. There's a vague recollection of something involving pizza, but I can't recall for sure what came next. After that trauma, it was a long time before I was able to walk into a bowling alley again.

Vegan Pizza

Preparation time: 15 minutes
Cooking time: 20 minutes
Serving size: 6

Ingredients:

4 Tbs. Olive oil
2 Yellow Onions, sliced
1 Garlic head, sliced
4 oz. Olives, ripe, sliced
8 oz. Crimini mushrooms, sliced
4 sprigs Basil, fresh, sliced
½ C. Tomato sauce
4 oz. Sundried tomatoes

1 Bell pepper, green - julienne sliced
1 Bell pepper, red – julienne sliced
¼ C. Pepperoncini
¼ C. Jalapeno peppers
1 Tbs. Oregano
1 Pizza dough or flatbread

Directions:

Heat oven to 375 degrees. Saute the vegetables in a bit of olive oil—all vegetables except the peppers, Pepperoncini, and olives. Leave a sprig of basil to add just before placing the pizza in the oven.

Roll out the dough in a round or rectangle if you prefer to 1/2 to 1 inch thickness. Place the dough on a cookie sheet. Much of the preparation time is spent slicing the vegetables unless you use food processor features. In that case your prep time is much shorter. Spread the dough with tomato sauce to cover all but the edges. Then in layers add the sautéed vegetables in the order you prefer. Add the set aside fresh basil. Drizzle olive oil to top the vegetables and coat the dough edge with oil. Place the pizza in the heated oven and bake until the crust edge turns light brown and vegetables appear heated through.

Serve:

Remove baked pizza from oven. Let set for 2 minutes before slicing in pie shaped triangles.

By now you see that my preferred cooking processes are sautéing, or roasting. I find they bring out the best flavors of the vegetables. Roasting is an especially effective process in that it cooks the vegetables from the inside to the outer layers. In doing so, I find it awakens flavors that isn't possible using any other cooking method.

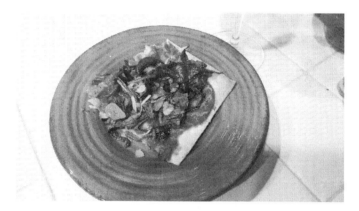

Roasted Root Vegetables

Preparation time: 30 minutes
Cooking time: 2 hours
Serving size: 6

Ingredients:

4 Tbs. Olive oil
2 Yellow Onions, quartered
4 Rainbow Carrots, quartered
1 Garlic head, whole
1 Rutabaga, large, quartered
1 White potato, large, quartered
1 Sweet potato, large, quartered
4 Celery stalks, cut crossways in
  1 inch pieces

2 Parsnips, quartered
2 Fennel bulbs, whole [fennel
  seeds are an option]
3 Beets, cut in half with greens
  removed
1 Tsp. cardamom
1 Tsp. coriander
½ C. Vegetable stock, organic
  low-sodium

Directions:

Heat oven to 375 degrees.

To prepare the vegetables – using a vegetable scrubber, clean the root vegetables to remove any excess dirt. Remove the ends from carrots, rutabaga, parsnips and beets. Remove the outer covering of the onion and the garlic. Separate each garlic clove and remove any remaining outer covering. Greens from the beets may be removed from the stem, cleaned and stored for use in other dishes later. Remove the bottom end of the fennel bulbs. Stalks and leaves of the fennel may be cut away from the bulb and roasted with the other vegetables. With the vegetables washed and the ends removed, they are now ready to coat with olive oil. Use just enough to cover the vegetable.

Cut the onions, potatoes, and rutabaga into quarters. Cut the carrots and parsnips in half length-wise, then cut in half width-wise. Cut the beets in half. Place the celery first then root vegetables in a roasting or baking dish arranged with the outer-side turned up in the dish. The outer-side is tougher and takes longer to cook until tender. Add the cloves of garlic making sure all the vegetables have contact with the garlic. Drizzle more olive oil over the vegetables in the dish. Sprinkle the cardamom and coriander over all the vegetables. Add vegetable broth to cover the bottom of the dish. Cover the dish with aluminum foil if there's no dish or pan top.

Place the dish in a pre-heated oven of 375 degrees and roast for about 90 minutes to 2 hours until all the root vegetables are fork tender.

About 30 minutes into the roasting your kitchen will be filled with the aromas of the vegetables, and seasoning combination as the broth steams through the vegetables mixing with their own juices. The pungent rutabaga and parsnip against the sweetness of carrots, beets and sweet potato. The smells are punctuated with cardamom and coriander. The onions, garlic, and the licorice scent of the fennel together makes for a syncopation that will have your taste buds dancing with anticipation to taste.

If you've never had fresh roasted red beets before you should know that the color runs and is released in the cooking process. It will affect the other vegetables. The color will also appear in your own body's elimination products, if you know what I mean. So, don't be alarmed.

HOLIDAY DISHES

Pumpkin Soup

Preparation time: 1 hour
Cooking time: 45 minutes
Serving size: 6

Ingredients:

1 Tbs. Olive oil
½ Onion, diced
½ Sweet Pumpkin, peeled and cubed
4 Cloves garlic, minced

1 Tbs. ginger, minced
6 sprigs of parsley
4-5 cups Vegetable stock
½ - 1 Cup Coconut Milk
¼ C. Almonds, sliced

Directions:

Heat oil in pan over medium heat; add onion and cook for a few minutes until the onion is translucent. Add pumpkin and garlic and continue to cook for a few minutes. Add ginger and vegetable broth. Bring the mixture to a boil. Reduce heat to low and simmer until pumpkin is tender and can be pierced with a fork. Puree the soup in a blender or food processor (in batches) and return to the pan. Add coconut milk and simmer for another minute or two.

Serve:

Ladle the soup in a bowl. Garnish with almonds and a bit of parsley.

Oyster Dressing

Preparation time: 45 minutes
Cooking time: 30 minutes
Serving size: 4-6 servings

Ingredients:

1 pt. Oysters and liquid
2 Tbs. Olive Oil
2 C. Yellow Onion, chopped
2 C. Celery, chopped
½ Tsp. Cayenne pepper
3 Bay leaves

1 Tbs. Garlic, minced
¼ C. Parsley, finely chopped
1 C. Water
¼ C. Green onion, chopped
4 C. French bread, cubed 1-inch

Directions:

Preheat oven to 375 degrees; Olive Oil 9 1/2 X 11 baking dish; Drain Oysters; Reserve oyster liquid. Heat oil in a large skillet over medium-high heat; add onions, celery, and cayenne pepper; Sauté for 5 minutes or until soft. Add bay leaves, garlic and parsley; Sauté for 1 minute; Add water and cook for 2 minutes stirring constantly. Add green onions oyster liquid and bread cubes. Stir to mix well and remove from the heat.

In a large mixing bowl combine the bread and vegetable mixture with oysters. Stir with a wooden spoon to mix thoroughly. Pour the mixture into a baking dish and bake for 1 hour or until bubbly and golden brown. Remove the bay leaves before serving.

If the dressing is to be used to stuff mushrooms, do not pour the mixture into a baking dish to bake. Set the mixture aside until the mushrooms are ready to stuff.

Cornbread Dressing

Preparation time: 30 minutes
Cooking time: 45 minutes
Serving size: 8-10

Ingredients:

2 Celery stalks
1 Onion, yellow (large)
2 Cornbread mix boxes
2 Eggs (egg substitute)
1¼ C. Almond or Cashew milk
½ Loaf white bread crumbs

¼ C. Thyme, fresh
¼ C. Sage, fresh
2 Tbs. Black Pepper, ground
4 Tbs. non-dairy butter
8 oz. Vegetable stock, warmed

Directions:

Preheat oven to 350 degrees. Coat a 9 X 11 baking dish with oil to prevent cornbread mixture from sticking to the dish.

Prepare the cornbread to start. It takes a bit of preparation. For convenience, I use cornbread mix. Follow directions on the box using non-dairy ingredients. Purists may make cornbread from scratch. There's a recipe in another section of this book. If making cornbread from scratch add another half hour to the preparation time. The cornbread mix usually takes about 5 minutes to mix and 20 minutes to bake. Once baked, let the cornbread cool another 15 minutes or so. While the cornbread is baking, the other dressing ingredients can be prepared.

Remove leaves from the celery stalks and put aside for use in soap or stews later. As I may have stated previously, I believe in using every bit of food for a nearly zero ecological footprint. Cut celery stalks in half length-wise. Then slice them in bite-sized pieces width-wise so they're shaped like half- moons. Place the cut celery in a large mixing bowl. Dice the onion, crumble the white bread into the bowl if they aren't already crumbled. Add the cornbread and seasonings. Blend all the ingredients well. Heat the vegetable stock until warm. Add non-dairy butter to the bowl ingredients, then pour the warmed vegetable stock over all and blend. When all the ingredients are well blended and moist, spoon the mixture into 9 X 11 baking dish. For moist cornbread dressing, cover the dish and place in a 350 degree oven for about 30 minutes. For cornbread with a crisp top, bake uncovered for about 30 minutes.

This dish can be prepared, up to the baking step, a day ahead. In fact it's best to do so to allow all the herbs and spices to fuse. On the meal-serving day, allow about 30 minutes for the dressing to bake.

Meats tend to be the centerpiece of most holiday or festive occasion traditions. The following recipe is a hearty substitute for holiday meats.

Stuffed Winter Squash

Preparation time: 45 minutes
Cooking time: 1 hour
Serving size: 6-8

Ingredients:

1 – Squash, large (acorn, butternut, hubbard, kabocha (has the texture and taste of sweet potato), or turban]
1 C. Quinoa, tri-colored
2¾ C. Vegetable stock
½ Onion, yellow or brown
2 Tbs. (heaping) Garlic, minced
2 Celery stalks
3 Carrots, diced
¼ C. Chives, chopped
½ C. Chestnuts
½ Tsp. Thyme (sage), fresh
1 C. Corn, organic (optional)
2 Tbs. Black Pepper, ground
½ C. Red onion
1 C. Crimini mushrooms
½ C. Orange juice

Directions:

This recipe requires two key steps, but it's worth it.

Step 1: Preparing the Squash: I use kabocha squash. I like the texture and taste. Rinse the squash. Cut it and remove seeds, strings (if any) to create an empty cavity; either cut an opening at the top pumpkin- like or in half. Using olive oil, oil the squash exterior and place in a shallow baking dish with 1/4 inch of orange juice. Bake with the flesh side down for about 30 minutes or until a fork can partially penetrate the squash at 375 degrees. Remove from oven and let stand until stuffing is ready.

Step 2: Preparing the stuffing: Cook the quinoa in 2 cups of vegetable stock. Following directions on the package, simmer the quinoa until all the liquid is absorbed and set aside. Sauté the mushrooms in a pan until golden brown. Meanwhile, in a large bowl combine onions, celery, chestnuts, carrots, sage, and garlic. Fold in cooled quinoa, and mushrooms. Add vegetable stock, thyme and black pepper. Mix ingredients thoroughly. Fill the squash cavity with the stuffing mixture, replace the squash lid for cover and return the squash to the oven. Bake for another 30 minutes or until the squash is tender. Remove from oven let stand for 5 minutes.

Serve:

Slice squash and plate with stuffing.

Collard Greens and Red Pepper Holiday Wreath

Preparation time: 15 minutes
Cooking time: 45 minutes
Serving size: 4

Ingredients:

3 Tbs. Vegetable stock
12 C. Collard Greens
4 Tsp. Lemon Juice or Balsamic
vinegar
1 Tbs. Nutmeg

2 Tsp. Red peppers, dried
crushed
1 Tbs. Garlic, minced
½ C. Sweet Red peppers, pickled
1 Tbs. Olive oil, extra virgin

Directions:

In a sauce pan, heat olive oil. Place greens, garlic, nutmeg, and crushed red peppers into the pan and cook. Add vegetable stock to keep the greens from sticking to pan. Cook the greens until tender. Drain excess liquid. In a large bowl, add lemon juice to greens stir with fork to coat. Arrange greens on a warm plate to create a wreath with space in the center. Arrange pickled red pepper on surface of the wreath as a bow and serve.

Part 4

Plant–based Cooking & My Health Outcomes

Having come this far sharing my life experiences and meals with you, I feel close enough to share my personal medical records since adopting a plant-based diet. I share this information to illustrate how effective this approach is to improved health. The tables below are readings from blood work and weight covering more than one year from 2014 to September 2015.

I actually began this nutritional journey in the fall of 2013. You'll see that by February 2014, six months later, I still had readings higher than the standard range. I was already on blood pressure medication—100 mg of Atenolol and 10 mg Lisinopril. By February 2014, my doctor prescribed 20 mg of Simvastatin to lower my cholesterol and keep my 63-year-old arteries open. I finally filled the prescription after continuous prodding by the doctor's office.

Kaiser Permanente, my health plan, uses a progressive system for monitoring patient activity. Office visits, lab work—blood and x-rays, pharmacy, hospital are all on one campus and electronically connected. Although I filled the prescription, I never took the drug. I disclosed this each time I saw my doctor, stating I wanted to reduce my cholesterol on my own. What you see in the chart is the outcome of that decision and my changed dietary behavior.

Test Name	2/22/2014	9/4/2015	Standard Range
Cholesterol	249	169	<= 199 mg/dl
Cholesterol/High Density Lipoprotein	6.7	4.6	<= 4.2
Cholesterol, Non-HDL	212	132	
HDL	37	37	<= 40 mg/dl
LDL, calculated	165	99	<= 99 mg/dl
Triglyceride	235	166	<= 149 mg/dl
Glucose, Fasting	95	88	70-99 mg/dl

Measure	1/28/2014	9/4/2015	Standard Range
Weight	172	167	122 - 164
BMI	26.16	25.48	18.5 - 24.9
Height	5' 8"	5' 8"	

The nurse in my doctor's office called to relay the lab results. As she finished giving me the cholesterol readings, she asked in a surprised, higher than usual pitch voice, how did you do that?! I told her, "I became a Pescaterian." She asked what that was. When I told her she said, keep it up. You're doing great! My doctor emailed a response to a question about my results and wrote, great work! They seemed genuinely surprised that a patient could take control of their health in this way with such positive outcomes. It can be done. If I can do it, anyone can.

From these lipid panel readings I am no longer required to take the Simvastatin for cholesterol. In April 2011 I was at my heaviest weighing 188 lbs. My weight and Body Mass Index (BMI) numbers are now going in the right direction—down. To maintain or even lower these encouraging readings, this dietary change is necessary for my lifetime, not just for a point-in-time. I can never go back to eating the way I used to if I want to have better health and ultimately a better quality of life as I grow older.

Epilogue

The volume of information from credible sources about what foods or diets are good for you and what isn't is dizzying. New information is revealed daily. Some new information can contradict that from the day before. It gets very confusing. I hope this book helps to distill available information to a point of clarifying some of the confusion or at least stir up enough curiosity to spur your own investigation. It is my hope that your take-away messages include that it isn't necessary to attend culinary school or have a medical degree to prepare tasty, health sustaining foods that are soul inspired, age-defying, and life-supporting. This book should also underscore the importance of:

Paying attention to your body and how it reacts to food

You are the best judge of your health and what food works for you. Don't ignore or dismiss the way you feel after eating. Doing so may mean you miss signs and signals of what your body needs to function properly. It is that information you will need to convey to your doctor if it becomes necessary. While there may be some genetic predisposition to food reactions, and health conditions, we are individually unique beings and our bodies respond differently to different foods.

Change your relationship with food

Food shouldn't be taken for granted. It isn't just to satisfy hunger. Food shouldn't be an escape from emotional upsets or social gaps. Food provides the energy we need to function. It's like gasoline is to a car. Treat your body as well as you treat your car. Its maintenance depends on what you feed it. Your body is a temple, a sacred vessel. To a certain extent, our body comes equipped to heal itself, if we let it, given an adequate food supply. Remember it was Hippocrates, the father of medicine, who is quoted as saying, "Let food be thy medicine and medicine be thy food." Be more thoughtful about what you consume. Only eat the best quality food—fresh, wholesome, nutritionally sound.

Question what's in our food and safe to consume

With all the uncertainty about what's in our food, particularly meats, we must become more knowledgeable about food production, processing, and content. Beef is regularly recalled due to E. coli and other sanitation concerns; poultry doesn't seem to be any safer with salmonella; not to mention the use of antibiotics, growth hormone injections and the like. That's not to say that plant foods are guaranteed safe. I remember a spinach recall several years ago.

A regional fast food restaurant chain promotes the fact that they now have a burger that's "all natural," "made with grass-fed beef, no-hormone injections, and no-antibiotics." It makes you wonder what's in the burgers they sell that are not "all natural." Then there's the GMO or genetically modified organism controversy over food with altered DNA. There's no conclusive information about the long-term effects on human health this process might have. Without GMO labeling, food production, processing information is incomplete effectively denying our ability to make fully informed food consumption decisions. We must hold regulatory agencies and public officials accountable for this.

Fearless recipe experimentation

Cooking is mostly instinctive and experimental. Be fearless! Don't be afraid to experiment with seasoning, food preparation, and a plant-based diet. You can transition into a plant-based diet gradually. Select one day a week to go meatless. Add days until you are meatless every day of the week.

The more you experiment, the more you will discover new "flavor profiles" and different food pairings and combinations that have never before been done.

It isn't disrespectful to your cultural or family traditions to switch out meat for legumes or nuts, to substitute nutrient-poor ingredients for those that are nutrient rich or to adopt different cooking methods.

It illustrates homage to the basic recipe while recognizing health concerns. It simultaneously shows respect for your body temple and family heritage.

Food transit and elimination

Changing your diet from essentially meat and potatoes to predominately plant food products will be quite a change to your gastrointestinal system. Your food transit time will increase. It may mean much more elimination than you're used to but don't let that frighten you.

There may be more flatulence and more poop. That may make some really uncomfortable, but it is better to have the food transiting swiftly through your system rather than festering inside and turning into something harmful to your health. As with anything, once your system becomes accustomed to the change, it won't feel so unusual and uncomfortable. And in the long-term, it's better for your health.

Change your relationship with your doctor. Enlist her as part of your health team.

Your doctor has professional training. But she can only apply her training based on information you provide about your condition and history to assess the condition you present. You should work in collaboration, conjunction and consultation with a healthcare professional in a spirit of mutual respect. Your doctor should be willing to listen to you and respect your opinion and values. That may mean changing doctors for one more compatible with you.

Appendices

Appendix A.

Tomato sauce

Ingredients:

Tomatoes – bushel basket

Fresh, unprocessed food is always best. If you can, making your own rather than buying and stocking canned tomato sauce is preferred.

You'll need a bushel of tomatoes—combination beefsteak, and Roma—that will yield approximately 8- quarts of tomato sauce. The beefsteak variety gives the sauce a tangy flavor. The tang is balanced by the sweetness of the Roma tomatoes. Removing the skin and seeds from the tomato is the key to making tomato sauce.

The good stuff where most nutrients lie is just under the skin of any fruit or vegetable. To retain the most nutrients, you want to steam the skin away rather than cut it off. To steam tomatoes, place them in an 8-quart sauce pan with just enough water to cover the pan's bottom. Place the pan over high flame until the water begins to bubble. Turn down the flame and allow the tomatoes to sweat in the heated water. When the heat causes the skin to tear away from the flesh of the tomato, turn off the flame and allow the tomatoes to rest and cool. Once they've cooled, it is easier to remove the skin and discard it. To remove the seeds, strain the tomatoes through a sifter.

Once the skin and seeds are removed the tomatoes are ready to boil. As you will see, additional water isn't necessary. Tomatoes generate enough liquid on their own. Turn the flame to high and allow the tomatoes to boil. In addition to being full of water, tomatoes are naturally salty. There is no need to add salt. If you choose to you can add dried, ground herbs like basil, oregano, thyme, and cumin. You may also decide to add fresh minced or sliced garlic. Adding the seasonings at this time will give them the chance to blend into the sauce making it more flavorful. When the tomatoes have a solid boil, turn the flame to low and let them simmer down to a thick consistency. This could take 3-4 hours.

This process of making tomato sauce is a perfect activity for a cold winter day. It will warm your house and fill the air with a salivating aroma.

Appendix B.

Garlic (herb) butter

Ingredients:

Non-dairy butter tub
Garlic, fresh head
Herbs – parsley, oregano, basil, etc. – fresh or dried

I like to have seasoned butter on hand to add to a recipe and give it richness.

I add my favorite herbs or garlic or both to butter. I start with a tub of non-dairy "butter." The non-animal product kind that has no cholesterol, non-GMO, etc. Let the tub sit at room temperature to soften for at least five hours. Meanwhile, you prepare the herbs you want to add. Dried herbs are preferred for their longer shelf life of one to three months. You can buy fresh herbs and dry them yourself or buy them dried.

To dry fresh herbs. Remove any stems. Spread them on a cookie sheet and place in an oven heated to 350 degrees. Turn the oven off and place the herb-filled cookie sheet inside the oven. When the herbs are crisp, remove them from the oven and place them between waxed paper to crumble them with a rolling pin. Set the herb aside until the butter is softened to fold them in.

For garlic butter, I roast several garlic heads in their hulls. Once roasted, squeeze the garlic from each clove into softened butter and stir until the garlic is fulling incorporated. Garlic butter adds another layer of flavor to any dish that has garlic as an ingredient for those of us who love garlic. I always say you can never have too much.

Herbs I use to make herb butter most are:

- Basil
- Oregano
- Parsley
- Dill

I sometimes stir herbs into garlic butter to add great flavor to almost any dish.

You can make butter specific to a particular cuisine. For example, basil and oregano butter go well in dishes with a tomato-sauce base. Dill butter adds flavor to fish and seafood dishes.

Appendix C.

Nut Butter

Ingredients:

1½ lbs. Nuts – almonds, cashews, filberts, etc.
⅓ C. Honey (optional)
Olive oil, extra virgin – by sight until smooth consistency is reached

This becomes a necessity if you're allergic to peanuts, like I am. While I'd prefer not to have to make it, making my own nut butter is the only alternative since some ready-made nut butters—almonds, cashews, pecans, etc. are manufactured in facilities where peanuts are also processed so you risk exposure.

Now more than ever you will need to use the food processor. It's really very easy with a food processor. Pour nuts of your choice into the food processor container cup. A pound of nuts yields about 2 cups of butter. Slowly pour olive oil through the liquid opening while grinding the nuts until they reach a buttery consistency. If you wish, pour in honey to enhance the flavor. Store the nut butter at room temperature in an air tight container. When it sits for a while, the oil may rise and separate from the nut paste. You will need to stir it before using it as a spread.

Appendix D.

Glossary

- ***Al dente*** – Cooked enough to retain a firm texture.
- ***Baby-Boomers*** – persons born between 1946 and 1964.
- ***Caramelize*** – a cooking method that produces sweetness in a food product.
- ***Generation X or Gen X*** – Persons born between 1965 and 1979.
- ***Genetically Modified Organism (GMO)*** – Foods produced with changes to their DNA using genetic engineering.
- ***Gluten*** – Elastic protein substance of wheat flour that binds dough.
- ***Gruel*** – a thin porridge.
- ***Mirepoix*** – a sautéed mixture of diced carrots, celery, and onions used as a base for soups, stews and sauces.
- ***Organic*** – Refers to how food products are grown using only substances derived from living organisms.
- ***Pescatarian*** – Diet where meat protein is derived from fish or seafood only.
- ***Vegan*** – Diet that excludes all animal products including dairy.
- ***Vegetarian*** – Diet that excludes meat from any living creature; but includes dairy.
- ***Scratch cooking*** – Method of cooking where the dish is completely made by hand with no prepared ingredients.

Physical Conditions

- ***Anorexia Nervosa*** – A serious eating disorder characterized by a pathological fear of weight gain leading to faulty eating patterns, malnutrition, and excessive weight loss.
- ***Body mass index (BMI)*** – A measure of body fat based on height and weight that applies to adult men and women, according to the National Institutes of Health.

- *Heart Murmur* – The sound the blood makes passing through valves of the heart. Most are innocent, but some can be associated with damaged or overworked heart valves.

- *Pulmonary Embolism* – Blockage of a main or branch artery of the lungs by a substance that has traveled from somewhere else in the body.

Acknowledgments

This book is the sum total of my experiences and acquired knowledge. It was created out of a compulsion to share the wisdom I've gained on food and the health connection over the years. The intention is to contribute to the betterment of the human experience. It would not have been possible without the assistance and supreme support from a team of beings both seen and unseen.

Carl Large, my confidante, my inspiration, who encouraged me, gently cajoled, provided key information, listened actively, taught me patience, and brought his great sense of humor at just the right moments. I am most grateful. Without his bolstering, I might have fallen into a procrastination abyss.

My son and daughter-in-law, Habib and Liann Williams West provided great moral support. This GenX duo challenged me to provide the most relevant information that resonated with them. They spurred greater recipe variety and more stylized food photos.

My sisters Diane Houston and Barbara White have always been my backbone. Their words of encouragement to be authentic helped to usher forth relatable stories from our upbringing.

One impetus for this book came from Jana Hexter who urges *Wisdom Keepers* to emerge; pressing that now is the time for my knowledge and wisdom to be shared. Coral Crew-Noble introduced me to Jana and has been a source of encouragement for nearly 30 years.

Cynthia Oredugba, my life coach, was instrumental in generating practical exercises requiring that I dig deep to excavate pertinent experiences from my memory. Always positive, always insightful Cynthia was invaluable in helping me set targets and timelines for my writing progression.

I am forever grateful for the keen editorial feedback from creative writers Marcia Hardy and Janice Taylor. Marcia, also a prolific grant writer, cheered my writing style. Janice, a communications specialist, encouraged descriptions that brought the stories "to life"; she suggested a more readable structure and more efficient use of language.

I am appreciative of Lillian Lew, M.Ed., RDN who provided rich insight from her training as a registered dietician. Always eager to provide health education, I am lucky Lillian was available.

As to the unseen beings, my mother Tryphena and grandmother Annie for whom I attribute my drive, spurred my curiosity about our health history, and compassion for justice in food politics and elsewhere.

To my Aunt Ida and Uncle Joe from whom I am happy to have caught a contagious love of food and fun with cooking.

I am grateful to divine Spirit through which all things are possible. My meditation and centered-down thoughtfulness allowed me to tap into Spirit, unleash the gifts with which I was endowed, and act as its hand. In so doing, as in the words of an Agape* affirmation, we are able to *be an anchor point for the next stage of human evolution.*"

*Agape International Spiritual Center is a non-denominational community and practice that promotes new thought, ancient wisdom principles for self-realization and a transformational world. It is the place where the author receives her spiritual food.

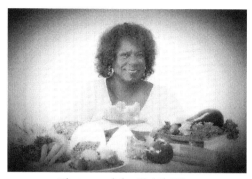

Photograph by Habib West

Gwendolyn Flynn *is a long-time champion of food as medicine. In her non-profit management position as a policy director with Community Health Councils, she led the development of food access policy strategy for more than a decade as a means of addressing preventable chronic diet-related disease in vulnerable Los Angeles populations. She knows first-hand the effects of food on health and since adopting a plant-based diet has had positive health outcomes. She studied nutrition and health as part of her Bachelor of Science degree at the State University of New York at Empire College. She is co-founder of SECONDS, a surplus food recovery and distribution non-profit. She is a mother, has two grandchildren and is a lifelong home cook. A resident of Los Angeles,* **Age-Defying, Soul Inspired, Plant-Based Cooking** *is her first book.*

Made in the USA
Middletown, DE
14 May 2018